TAMING ASTHMA and ALLERGY by CONTROLLING Your ENVIRONMENT

TAMING ASTHMA and ALLERGY by CONTROLLING Your ENVIRONMENT

A Guide for Patients

by

ROBERT A. WOOD, M.D.

Illustrations By I. Robert Wood, M.D.

Note to the Reader

While this book is designed to help you to better understand and deal with your allergies or asthma, it is not intended to be a substitute for the ongoing care of your own personal physician. The author and publisher therefore disclaim any responsibility for any adverse effects resulting from the information presented in this book and urge you to consult your physician before implementing any of the information contained herein.

Published by Asthma and Allergy Foundation of America,
Maryland Chapter, Inc.
Chester Building, Suite 321, 8600 LaSalle Road
Towson, Maryland 21286-2002

Library of Congress Catalog Card Number: 94-79901

ISBN 0-9643272-0-1

Text and Cover Design by Harry Rinehart

Manufactured in the United States of America

Second Printing

Acknowledgements

Although I am indebted to many individuals who helped to make this book possible, there are several who deserve special recognition.

Mr. John Riina, Executive Director of the Maryland Chapter of the Asthma and Allergy Foundation of America, came to me with the idea for this book and has since attended to every detail in its development. His interest and support have been invaluable.

I owe a great deal to all the researchers who have contributed to the science of allergy and environmental control. In particular, I would like to pay special thanks to Drs. Thomas Platts-Mills and Martin Chapman at the University of Virginia who have led the way in the study of indoor allergens.

I would like to thank my friend and mentor at Johns Hopkins, Dr. Peyton Eggleston, for all that he has done for me.

Finally, I owe special thanks to my family. My parents have always set a shining example for me, and my father, Dr. I. Robert Wood, even applied his exceptional talents as an artist to the illustrations in this book. Most of all, however, I am indebted to my wife, Dr. Renee Melly Wood, for her unyielding support and incredible patience.

Asthma and Allergy Foundation of America
Maryland Chapter
Chester Building, Suite 321
8600 LaSalle Road
Towson, Maryland 21286-2002
(410) 321-4710
E-mail: aafamd@bcpl.net
www.aafa-md.org

Asthma and Allergy Foundation of America
1125 15th Street, NW • Suite 502
Washington, DC 20005
(202) 466-7643 • (800) 727-8462

The Asthma and Allergy Foundation of America (AAFA) is dedicated to finding a cure for and controlling asthma and allergic diseases. AAFA serves the estimated 50 million Americans with asthma and allergic diseases through the support of research, patient and public education programs, public and governmental advocacy, and a network of chapters and support groups located throughout the nation.

The Asthma and Allergy Foundation of America's Maryland Chapter was founded in 1979 as a natural outgrowth of the needs of asthma and allergy patients. The Chapter is a member of the national Asthma and Allergy Foundation of America, serving Americans for more than 40 years.

Contents

Preface

More than forty million Americans suffer from allergies. For some people, allergies are nothing more than a mild inconvenience. For many others, however, allergies are a cause of serious illness. They are a major reason for missed school and work for both children and adults, and in some they can trigger severe, life-threatening reactions. If you or your child suffers from some form of allergic disease, you are well aware of the suffering that can be involved.

Most people use medications as their first line of defense in treating allergic disease. If these fail, they will most likely try avoidance measures and allergy shots. Fortunately, medical science has made tremendous advances in all areas of allergy treatment in recent years. Better and safer medications and more effective allergy shots are now available. Just as important, however, are the advances in our understanding of the allergens themselves and in developing more effective techniques of avoiding them.

Although you can never escape all of the allergens in your environment, you can do a great deal to reduce your exposure to most of them. It certainly seems most logical to try first to avoid the allergens that are causing your symptoms and then to use medications or allergy shots for the exposures that you cannot control. This book is about managing allergies and asthma through allergen avoidance, which we will also call *environmental control*. We will review the nature of allergic reactions, discuss the allergens themselves, and then concentrate on a logical approach to environmental control.

You can use this book in a variety of ways. I would encourage you to read it from cover to cover, if you have the time and energy to do so, so you will achieve maximum information and understanding. However, each section is designed to stand on its own to a large degree, and you can therefore pick and choose sections of particular interest. For example, if animal allergens are an important issue for you or your family, you could read that chapter first and still understand it without going through all of the preceding chapters. So take a look at the table of contents, read on, and enjoy!

PART 1

Introduction

CHAPTER 1

Case Histories

By way of introduction, I would like to tell you about some patients who have had great success in treating their allergies through environmental control. These patients have taught me a lot about allergy, environmental control, and even human nature. You need not be too concerned with the details—many of the allergens and environmental control measures mentioned here may be unfamiliar to you, but they will be explained in detail over the course of the book. My intent here is rather to introduce you to allergy through these personal stories.

Although I will cover them in more detail later, a few definitions might be helpful before you begin. An *allergy* is a general term that describes an abnormal reaction (sensitivity) to a substance that is normally tolerated without difficulty. The term *allergic* is used to describe an individual who has one or more allergies. An *allergen* refers to any foreign substance that induces an allergic reaction. *Allergic rhinitis* refers to an allergic reaction that involves the nose, and *asthma* is a condition that causes a narrowing of the airways in the lungs.

CASE 1: THE HIDDEN DUST MITE

Mary first came to see me when she was five years old. Her parents and pediatrician were concerned because she was having frequent asthma attacks that seemed to be growing more and more severe and would occur whenever she caught a cold. Medications would eventually work, but in the meantime Mary would typically suffer for several days, during which her parents often spent sleepless nights watching her breathe and debating whether or not they should take her to the hospital. Mary's asthma had become a dominant feature in their lives, and they lived in constant fear of her next attack. Fortunately, between her colds Mary's asthma seemed to disappear, leaving her happy and symptom free without medication.

There was nothing too remarkable about Mary's environment. The house was about eighty years old and was heated by hot water radiators. Mary slept in her own bedroom that had a hardwood floor with an area rug. Her bed had an ordinary innerspring mattress and box spring. She slept with a foam pillow and a down comforter, as well as several stuffed animals to keep her company. There seemed to be no problem with excess moisture or mold growth, and there were no pets in the home. Her parents would not allow anyone to smoke either in the house or in their car.

During her physical examination, Mary was a shy but delightful five year old. She appeared to be extremely healthy. Her nose was slightly congested, but her chest was entirely clear, and the remainder of her exam was completely normal.

I suggested to her parents that it might be a good idea to test Mary with some common allergens. Because her asthma showed no seasonal pattern, I explained that it would make sense to rule out allergies to the common indoor allergens. Moreover, because it takes a certain degree of exposure to become allergic, I also explained that it would be more likely for a young child like Mary to react to allergens to which she had been exposed on a year-round basis. Her parents were concerned that this testing was unnecessary. They had searched for possible triggering agents and could find none except for her frequent colds. They had decided, quite logically, that if she had allergies her symptoms would be apparent all the time, not just when she had colds.

They were also concerned that Mary would find the testing very unpleasant.

After some discussion, we decided to proceed with a limited number of skin tests. Mary was tested for allergy to dust mites, cockroaches, and molds. She tolerated the testing very well—she sat on her mother's lap and never even cried. She was found to be highly allergic to both of the common dust mites. On a scale of 0 to 4, she had what we would rate a 4-plus reaction.

I explained to her parents the possible significance of these results and recommended that they institute environmental controls for dust mites. Although they were still puzzled over how dust mites could be important since Mary wheezed only when she had a cold, they were determined to find any possible relief for their daughter. They were also particularly excited that there might be an option other than more medication. They immediately bought plastic covers for the mattress, box spring, and pillow and replaced the down comforter with a washable bedspread. They removed the stuffed animals and the area rug from Mary's bedroom.

Once these controls were in place, Mary's asthma improved dramatically. For the first time, she could get through most of her colds without having an asthma attack, and when she did develop symptoms, they were mild and easily controlled. The improvement has now continued for more than two years, and although Mary still has asthma, it no longer disrupts her life. Her parents have told me repeatedly that they feel as if they have been relieved of a tremendous burden.

Although this is not an altogether typical case of dust mite allergy, it is nevertheless very instructive. As the parents had assumed, the more characteristic case would have involved more persistent symptoms between attacks. Let me try to explain, however, how this case really is consistent with dust mite allergy and how it might even be just as common a story as the patient with obvious, uninterrupted symptoms.

We believe that Mary, and many other patients like her, develop a state of low grade inflammation (irritation with redness and swelling) in their airways because of their daily exposure to indoor allergens. The inflammation can be so mild that no outward symptoms are apparent. If you had been able to look down into Mary's lungs, however, you would have seen that the lining of her airways was slightly swollen and inflamed even when she appeared completely well. Although this allergic reaction did not produce persistent symptoms, it made her vulnerable to a more severe attack when she was exposed to an additional trigger such as a cold or other viral infection. Once this inflammation was relieved through allergen avoidance, she was finally able to withstand these other triggers without experiencing an asthma attack.

Because of cases like this, we only rely to a small degree on the history of symptoms upon exposure to indoor allergens. It may take allergy tests to define the problem more fully, and we therefore recommend that all patients who are having significant problems with asthma or allergies undergo allergy testing. Then we are able to implement appropriate environmental controls based on the test results and, as in the case of Mary, hope that our efforts will improve the patient's overall health and quality of life.

CASE 2: THE ALLERGIC NIGHTMARE

Thomas was three years old when I first met him in the allergy clinic. He had a history of asthma since infancy, and his symptoms were becoming more difficult to control as time passed. He had been admitted to the hospital four times the year before and had to be taken to the emergency room with an asthma attack at least once a month. These problems had persisted in spite of aggressive treatment with medications. Understandably, his family and his pediatrician were growing extremely concerned and frustrated.

In addition to his asthma, Thomas had persistent, severe nasal congestion. He was barely able to breathe through his nose and had even become very uncomfortable when trying to sleep. However, unlike most of us, who would experience this as a huge problem, Thomas and his family regarded it as minor compared with the severity of his asthma.

When I asked about Thomas's home environment, I learned that he lived with his mother, two siblings, a grandmother, two aunts, and several cousins in a three-bedroom row house in Baltimore. He shared a bed with his mother in a room in which an aunt and two cousins also slept. The bedroom had wall-to-wall carpeting, but the rest of the house had tile or wood floors. All of the adults smoked in the home, and his mother even smoked in bed with him. They frequently saw cockroaches, and two cats had free run of the house, often sleeping on Thomas's bed. Finally, the roof leaked, and mold grew on the walls of the bedroom, bathroom, and kitchen.

On physical examination, Thomas was found to be an active and playful little boy. He had obvious "allergic shiners"—dark circles around the eyes which are often seen in people with allergies. The lining of his nose was so swollen that his nasal passages were completely blocked on both sides. I heard mild wheezing when I listened to his chest.

On skin tests for the common indoor allergens, Thomas was highly allergic to dust mites, cockroaches, cats, and a variety of molds. Although I would have guessed that Thomas was allergic, the test results were surprising because children that age are rarely sensitive to so many different allergens.

As opposed to the more subtle case of Mary, it was clear that allergies were playing a major role in Thomas's problems. He was very allergic, was having persistent symptoms, and was obviously being exposed to several major allergens on a regular basis. But even though changes in the environment were desperately needed, the odds against bringing about those changes seemed almost overwhelming.

I decided that at least a few things were under our control and that it would be most logical to begin with those. I began by recommending that all cigarette smoking be stopped in the home. Thomas's mother agreed but warned that her mother absolutely would not. She (the grandmother) said that she had never seen Thomas get sick from cigarette smoke, so it therefore was not a problem. I tried to explain that any smoke exposure is extremely irritating to the lungs and could have devastating effects for a child like Thomas. I even wrote a note for Thomas to take home to his grandmother, but she replied that it was her house, and she would do as she pleased.

Next, I recommended that they remove the cats from the home. Although the family agreed that they would try to keep the cats out of Thomas's bedroom, his mother told me that if they got rid of them altogether the mice would take over the house. I realized that I had completely missed this when I had asked about their environment and went on to discover that they saw mice on a daily basis and that the cats were essential for their control. I then applied a skin test for mouse allergen and found that it too was strongly positive. The odds were growing even more overwhelming.

When we discussed dust mite and mold control, the mother agreed to get a plastic cover for their mattress and pillows. We were still left with a wall-to-wall carpet, however, and significant problems with moisture. She explained that their landlord was unwilling to fix the leaky roof, which made prospects for a significant reduction in either mite or mold exposure very slim. I recommended that she try to eliminate all of the areas of mold growth using a dilute bleach solution.

The last issue was the cockroaches. When we discussed this further, it really sounded as if they were an enormous problem. Apparently the house was teeming with them, as were the adjoining row homes. I recommended aggressive extermination and wrote a letter for her to give to her landlord. She warned me that he was unlikely to be helpful, and I had no reason to think otherwise.

Both the mother and I were pretty depressed by the end of our discussion. It seemed that we were faced with several insurmountable problems—the cats, the smoking, the mice, the cockroaches, and the moisture. And yet these environmental conditions were severely affecting Thomas's health. He had a severe form of asthma which was difficult to control and was even life threatening. It was clear that something had to be done.

We concluded that the family would have to find alternative housing. This is no simple process, however, even when a child's health is severely jeopardized. We began by sending letters to the housing authority but got no response. After about six months and a long battle that involved a disability determination for Thomas and help from a lawyer, the family found a new place to live. We would never have succeeded, however, had it not been for the mother's persistence and her willingness to work two jobs to earn extra income. During that six-month battle, Thomas remained ill and was hospitalized two more times in spite of intense medical therapy, including the regular use of steroids. Since the move, however, he has remained out of the hospital, has been easily maintained off steroids, and can even breathe through his nose! Although he still has serious asthma, he will hopefully never need to be hospitalized again and may no longer be at risk of dying from his disease.

CASE 3: THE CAT ALLERGIC FAMILY

This story begins with a cat lover named Jim. His family had owned cats while he was growing up, and, although he had developed some problems with allergic rhinitis (nasal allergy) by the time he was a teenager, he refused to believe that the cats could be playing any role. He should have become more suspicious when his symptoms disappeared when he went away to college and returned whenever he came home, but he either ignored that fact or decided it was not important. In reality, his symptoms were mild, and it was not necessarily inappropriate to ignore the possibility of cat allergy. However, when he finished college he took matters a step further and got two cats of his own. Although he still considered his symptoms to be relatively mild, he did find himself at the doctors more and more often with sinus infections. His doctor referred him to an allergist, but Jim decided not to go.

Along the way Jim met Susan. They began dating and were getting along fabulously except for one problem: Susan had grown up with asthma and knew she was extremely allergic to cats. Jim would clean his apartment feverishly before she would come over, but she would still grow uncomfortable after being there for any length of time. Jim even bought an air cleaner and hired a cleaning lady. As time passed, Susan seemed to be able to tolerate the cats a little better, and much to Jim's delight, she began to like them. A year or two later Jim and Susan decided to get married. After some debate, they decided that the cats would stay.

During their first year of marriage, Susan's asthma took a gradual turn for the worse. She required increasing doses of medication and was having symptoms almost every day. She would often wake up coughing and wheezing. Of note, she would also commonly wake up with the cats sleeping next to her! Jim continued to have frequent sinus infections. Finally, they both went to an allergist. Tests showed that they were both highly allergic to cats, and the allergist urged them to find a new home for their pets. After much discussion, they decided to keep the cats but to step up their efforts at environmental control. They tried to keep the cats out of the bedroom and kept the air cleaner running continuously. The allergist adjusted their medications and started them on allergy shots.

Over the next two years things stayed about the same. They read about some new research on washing cats and began to do that regularly. They felt that their medications were effective and thought that the allergy shots were helping. Actually, they were so fond of their cats that they were willing to overlook a great deal of illness and discomfort. Susan still had regular symptoms in spite of daily medication, and Jim was now seeing an ear, nose, and throat specialist for help with his recurrent sinus infections. He required frequent antibiotics and eventually even needed sinus surgery.

I first met Jim and Susan when they were expecting their first child. They came with specific concerns about how they might be able to prevent allergies and asthma in their child, given their very strong family history for these problems. They had heard that breast feeding would help and wondered what else they could do. I explained that breast feeding was an excellent idea and that it might be particularly beneficial if Susan avoided certain foods in her diet while nursing the baby. We also discussed different infant formulas and their effects on the development of allergy. Then I asked them about their home environment, particularly regarding pets and cigarette smokers. They assured me that neither of them smoked and then reluctantly told me about their two cats. I told them that I certainly could not predict the future but that if they really wanted to reduce their child's risk of developing allergy, they should find a new home for their cats. They said that was clearly out of the question. Although I could understand their decision in not taking this major step because of my theoretical concerns, I still stressed that all the breast feeding in the world might not overcome the adverse effects of early, intense exposure to cats.

I have now had the pleasure of taking care of their son Joshua for about two years. Unfortunately, his parents' "allergic genes" combined to produce a very allergic child. In spite of being breast fed, he began to show signs of eczema by the time he was two months old. His symptoms were fairly mild but gave some warning of what might be in store. I mentioned the cats again but with no more success. Susan and Jim still regarded that idea as "just a theory."

After this buildup I am sure you can guess what happened next. Joshua began wheezing when he was six months old and has required continuous asthma medication ever since. Although he did not have a positive allergy test to cats at that time, his parents were finally willing to give up their pets. They decided that even if the cats had not caused his early problems, odds were too high that they would contribute to future problems. It was an extremely difficult decision for them, but it was clearly the right one. That fact became even more obvious a year later, when Joshua had a strongly positive allergy test for cats!

Joshua's unfortunate problems had at least had one very positive outcome: both Jim and Susan have been dramatically healthier since the cats have been out of the house. Susan needs only occasional asthma medications, and Jim's nose and sinus problems have virtually disappeared.

This case helps to make a number of interesting and instructive points. The first has to do with the tremendous bond that people may develop with their pets. Here were two bright, educated adults who were chronically ill because of their ongoing exposure to cats, but who were unwilling to find a new home for them. Unfortunately, this is a very common scenario. It turns out that many people with animal allergies stubbornly refuse to remove the offending pets from their home. As in this case, it often takes a sick child to finally convince them to take that step, although some families will refuse to give up their pets even then.

A second point is that for some people, nothing short of removing the pet from the home will be sufficient. Although many less drastic techniques can reduce the allergen levels, they may not be even close to adequate for people with severe allergies. Even if bedroom doors are kept closed and efforts are made to reduce direct contact with the animals, these allergens travel widely within a home, ensuring that to some degree everyone will be exposed.

This case also demonstrates that although allergy shots may provide some relief for animal allergies, their ability to help significantly someone who is living with a pet is questionable. This is because the shots may not work well enough to provide adequate protection against the high levels of allergen to which animal owners are exposed on a daily basis. Shots are probably best reserved for those people who have only intermittent, unavoidable contact with cats or dogs. Why not try shots for people who keep their pets? The answer to that question is that the shots are expensive, inconvenient, and potentially dangerous: allergic reactions can occur in response to allergy shots, and in some cases these reactions can be severe. The bottom line for me is that once someone is having enough problems to consider shots, the pet should go!

One final point deserves note. As I will discuss later in the book, there is evidence that allergen avoidance early in life can provide a protective effect with regard to the future development of allergy and asthma. For a child such as Joshua, who has a strong family history of allergy and asthma, his parents should reduce his exposure to major allergens whenever possible. In this case, Jim and Susan were interested enough to come talk to me but were unwilling to make the real commitment to give up their cats. We will never know if Joshua would have still developed asthma if the cats had been removed, but I know I will always wonder.

CASE 4: THE IMPORTANCE OF IRRITANTS

Matthew was three years old when I first saw him to evaluate his persistent nasal congestion and recurrent ear and sinus infections. His parents reported that he had had these problems since infancy and that even then their pediatrician had warned them that he would be an allergic child. Matthew had taken a variety of antihistamines and decongestants without any success and frequently antibiotics in addition. He experienced his nasal congestion all year long, but his infections occurred most often in the fall and winter months. His doctors had placed tubes in his ears when he was just a year old, but they fell out when he was two. His parents were very reluctant to have him undergo surgery again to replace the tubes and wondered if something else could be done. Their pediatrician suggested that allergies might be contributing to Matthew's infections and referred the parents to me for consultation.

I found that Matthew was otherwise healthy. He was growing well and had never had any symptoms of asthma. He was an only child, and the family had no history of allergies or asthma. However, his mother did report that she had developed recurrent sinus infections and bronchitis as a young adult. She commented that she seemed to take antibiotics as often as Matthew.

Matthew and his parents lived in a three-year-old individual house in a rural area. The house had wall-to-wall carpeting and a heat pump. There were two dogs that were kept either outside the house or in the basement. Matthew slept in a regular bed with two favorite stuffed animals. There were no problems with excessive moisture or mold growth in the home. It turned out, however, that Matthew's father was a heavy smoker.

On physical examination, Matthew seemed to be a healthy boy, although both of his ears were mildly infected. His nose was very congested, and its lining was red and swollen. He had a yellow nasal discharge, which is much more consistent with infection or severe irritation than with allergy. His chest was clear, and the remainder of his exam was normal.

I performed allergy tests to a panel of common indoor allergens, including dust mites, dogs, cockroaches, and molds, which were the primary concern because of Matthew's age and because his symptoms were present year round. All of the tests were entirely negative. I examined a smear of his nasal secretions under the microscope; the material present was consistent with infection and showed no evidence of allergy.

I concluded that there was no evidence of an allergic cause for Matthew's problems. Because of his recurrent infections, I sent tests to examine his immune system; those results were also entirely normal. My final assessment was that the most likely cause for Matthew's problems was passive exposure to cigarette smoke, which was both irritating his nose and putting him at risk for repeated infections. I also learned that Matthew's father based his business in the home and that although he tried not to smoke around Matthew, he was constantly smoking somewhere in the house. Matthew's mother then commented that she found the cigarette smoke very irritating, both physically and emotionally, and that her problem sinusitis and bronchitis had actually not developed until after she was married. Needless to say, I gave her lots of new ammunition to use in her efforts to get her husband to quit smoking, at least in their home.

The last I knew, Matthew's father was still smoking but was only allowed to do so outside the house. He never really believed that his smoking had been responsible for his family's medical problems, but he had no choice but to change his behavior! Because of the existing damage, Matthew still had to undergo surgery to have tubes placed in his ears again. He is now doing extremely well, however, and no longer has any significant nasal congestion. His mother also reports that she no longer takes antibiotics since her escape from the intense smoke exposure.

Unfortunately, this is a very common scenario. Tobacco smoke is a potent irritant that is particularly damaging to children. It is a common cause of persistent nasal congestion in young children, and it puts exposed children at an increased risk of developing a variety of respiratory problems, including ear and sinus infections. Fortunately, Matthew did not develop any symptoms of asthma as will occur in some children with such exposure. It is also important to point out that this story might have had a very different ending if, as is often the case, both of Matthew's parents had been smokers who refused to believe that they were harming their child.

CASE 5: A VIRTUAL MOLD FACTORY

Timothy, a five year old, was brought to me a few months ago for evaluation of asthma, persistent nasal congestion, and recurrent sinus infections. He had been healthy until he was about three, when his parents noticed that he developed increasing nasal congestion. It had grown so severe that Tim could barely breathe through his nose, and he was having difficulty sleeping. The congestion was present year round with some worsening during the spring, summer, and fall. His parents tried several different allergy medications, but none seemed to help. About once a month Tim would also develop a sinus infection, usually accompanied by a thick green nasal discharge and a severe cough, particularly at night. His cough was so intense that his pediatrician felt he might have asthma and therefore placed him on a variety of asthma medications as well.

Tim's medical history was otherwise unremarkable. The family history was positive for allergic rhinitis in Tim's mother and two of her sisters. Tim had one brother who did not seem to have any problems with asthma or allergies.

Tim lived with his mother and brother in a twenty-year-old individual home. He slept in his own bedroom with a few stuffed animals. The room had wall-to-wall carpeting. His mother ran a humidifier in Tim's bedroom nightly because it seemed to relieve his congestion. The house had a gas furnace with forced air heat and a central humidifier. There was no air conditioning, but the family used window fans during hot weather. There were no pets or smokers in the home. Finally, they reported that the basement was damp and had a musty smell.

Tim's physical examination was noteworthy only for severe nasal congestion. The lining of his nose was very pale and swollen, which is typical of allergic rhinitis, and he had a profuse clear nasal discharge. His chest was clear, and the rest of his exam was normal.

I applied skin tests for both indoor and outdoor allergens. I found Tim to be mildly allergic to dust mites, grass, and ragweed and severely allergic to several types of common indoor and outdoor molds.

I explained to Tim's mother that he had severe allergic rhinitis that was related to both indoor and outdoor allergens. I further explained that it was likely that his allergy to indoor molds was the major cause of his persistent, year-round congestion. When I told her this, she said that she was not surprised because her basement was not just damp, it was wet and moldy. She went on to explain that the former owner of the house had grown marijuana in the basement and that the entire floor had been covered with a layer of dirt! She had done her best to clean things up, but the basement had remained very damp, and she had eventually covered the cement floor with carpeting. I then also learned that Tim's symptoms had begun to appear about six months after the family had moved into this house!

I told Tim's mother that it would take lots of work to reduce the mold growth in her house and that I was not even sure it could ever be sufficiently free of mold for Tim to live there comfortably. But we decided it was certainly worth a try and outlined a program that would require aggressive dehumidification and a great deal of cleaning. First, both humidifiers were turned off; extra moisture was the last thing that was needed. Second, Tim's mother purchased a high quality dehumidifier for the basement and kept it running continuously. I felt strongly that an air conditioner would also help, and although she did not have the money to buy one right away, she started to look into ways to fund it before the next summer. Next, she removed the carpet that she had placed over the cement floor in the basement. Finally, she put together a cleaning crew of several friends and relatives to help her scrub the house from top to bottom with a potent mix of water and bleach.

We started Tim on some new medications, and, with the environmental control measures in place, he has been doing very well. He has not needed any more asthma medication and has been able to stay off antibiotics. When they came in for a follow-up visit, Tim's nose looked much better, and his mother was rightfully proud of the steps she had taken to restore his health.

SUMMARY

I have chosen these cases to emphasize not just the potential adverse effects of environmental allergens and irritants on our health, but also the valuable role that environmental control and allergen avoidance can play in the treatment of patients with allergy and asthma. Because these cases are all success stories, they are not necessarily representative. For a variety of reasons, we have to face many failures along with our successes. Although the failures can be the result of limited finances or a home environment beyond repair, they are often due to a lack of understanding or a refusal to recognize the dangers of household pets or cigarette smoke. Hopefully, the successes reported here will encourage you to read on and learn more about allergies and environmental control.

PART 2

Allergies
and Allergens

CHAPTER 2

What Is an Allergy?

The word *allergy* is one of the most common medical terms used in everyday conversation. Physicians and patients alike blame allergies for a host of medical problems. In addition to well defined allergic diseases such as hay fever and asthma, symptoms as varied as headaches, stomach aches, and hyperactivity are also commonly attributed to an allergy. However, although allergies are indeed extremely common and some true allergies may even be overlooked, much that is called allergy is actually not allergy at all. We will therefore begin with a few definitions and examples of allergic diseases so that we can proceed with a common understanding of the term.

The word *allergy* comes from the Greek *allos,* which means *other*. Baron Clemens von Pirquet coined the term in 1906 to describe virtually any "altered reaction" within the immune system. By this original definition, these reactions could have been either harmful or beneficial to the body. Today, we define *allergy* as an abnormal sensitivity to a substance that most people can tolerate without difficulty. For example, most people experience no reaction to pollen, whereas persons with allergic rhinitis may react intensely after even a brief exposure. We now view this sensitivity as involving only certain specific parts of the immune system. A good synonym for *allergy* would be *hypersensitivity*, although that is a somewhat more general term.

The process by which one becomes allergic continues to be a subject of active research and debate. By definition, the process begins with a period of sensitization, during which repeated exposures to an allergen activate the immune system in some (susceptible) individuals. Although all of the details are still not well understood, whether or not someone becomes allergic depends on both genetic and environmental factors. For example, someone with a strong family history of allergy is far more likely to become allergic than someone with no such family history. According to current estimates, a child with one allergic parent has a 30 to 50 percent chance of developing allergies, while if both parents are allergic the odds rise to 60 to 80 percent.

In addition to genetics, the environment also appears to play a significant role in the development of allergy. Studies of identical twins best demonstrate the powerful role of these "nongenetic" factors. Despite their identical genetic makeup, only 25 to 50 percent of identical twins will acquire the same allergies or the same allergic disease. These differences are presumed to result primarily from different environmental exposures. Someone who is exposed over time to high levels of a particular allergen is more likely to become sensitive to that allergen than is someone with less exposure. For example, it has clearly been shown that exposure to high levels of dust mites early in life dramatically increases the chance of becoming dust mite allergic later in life. The odds are then increased further if there is a family history of allergy. On the other hand, some people seem to be virtually incapable of developing allergies no matter how intense the exposure.

Remarkably, this period of sensitization may last anywhere from weeks to decades. One person may develop a food allergy in the first few weeks of life, whereas another may not become sensitized until late in adulthood. With inhalant allergens, such as pollens and molds, most people become sensitized only after several years of exposure. The rate at which this process occurs probably also depends on both genetic and environmental factors. Exposure to certain non-specific irritants, particularly cigarette smoke, may also accelerate this process.

During the period of sensitization, the body produces specific *antibodies* against one or more of the allergens to which it has been exposed. Antibodies are chemicals that are produced by B lymphocytes, a type of white blood cell which makes up part of the immune system. The body produces a great variety of different antibodies in response to many outside stimuli. For example, specific antibodies are produced in response to immunizations or infections to protect the body against future infection.

Antibodies belong to a more general class of chemicals in the body called *immunoglobulins.* There are five major classes of immunoglobulins (abbreviated Ig): IgA, IgM, IgG, IgD, and IgE. Each different class of immunoglobulin has different functions in the body, and the antibodies that cause allergic reactions belong to the IgE class. During the process of sensitization, specific IgE antibodies are therefore produced against specific allergens. People only become sensitized to some of the allergens to which they are exposed, and subsequent allergic reactions will then occur only upon reexposure to those allergens against which specific IgE antibodies have been produced. Thus, one person may become allergic only to cats, whereas another may become allergic to a whole range of allergens. The reasons for these individual differences again lie in a combination of genetic and environmental factors that are still poorly understood.

Once a person has become sensitized to a particular allergen, he or she is at risk of developing allergic symptoms with each exposure to that allergen. Low levels of exposure might lead to only mild symptoms, whereas high levels of exposure may produce more immediate and severe symptoms. It also appears that many people become "primed" after repeated exposures, as would occur in a typical pollen season. When that happens, reactivity is increased such that lower and lower levels of exposure may produce increasingly severe symptoms.

Specific patterns of response are difficult or even impossible to predict over time, however. One person may grow worse with every season, and another may "outgrow" his or her symptoms over time. It is very common for children to display worsening symptoms with each year of added exposure. Allergies then tend to peak in number and severity in early adulthood.

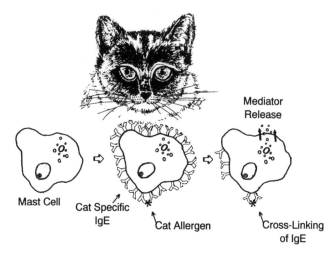

How an allergic reaction occurs

As shown in the accompanying diagram, the allergic reaction itself follows a regular sequence of events. First, the IgE antibodies that were produced in response to a given allergen attach themselves to the surface of the body's main allergy cells, called *mast cells* and *basophils.* Mast cells are located in the skin, nose, lungs, and gastrointestinal tract; basophils are found mainly in the blood. Because of their location, mast cells are ideally situated to come into contact with the allergens that enter the body, and they in turn make it possible for these allergens to come into contact with the IgE antibodies that lie on their surface. An allergic reaction will then be initiated if the arriving allergen finds on the mast cells specific IgE antibodies that have been produced because of prior exposures to that allergen. When enough allergen is present to connect two adjacent IgE molecules (called *cross-linking*), the mast cell releases a variety of chemicals that are referred to as *mediators.*

These mediators, the best known of which is histamine, cause many of the common allergic symptoms with which we are all familiar, such as sneezing, runny nose, itching, and wheezing. Since all of this takes place very quickly, these symptoms can begin within minutes of exposure to the allergen. In addition, however, it is now also clear that some mediators have effects that are not seen for hours after the initial reaction. These mediators cause other kinds of blood cells, including basophils and another type of white blood cell called *eosinophils*, to come to the site of the initial reaction, causing an even more intense response. These so-called *late phase reactions* are important because they produce swelling and inflammation that can be more severe and more difficult to treat than the initial reaction. We are now convinced that these late reactions, which occur hours after the allergen exposure, are a major cause of many chronic allergic symptoms, including asthma.

COMMON ALLERGIC DISEASES

I would like to take a moment to describe the common allergic diseases and their symptoms. Our emphasis will be on inhalant allergies, which mainly affect the nose (allergic rhinitis), the eyes (allergic conjunctivitis), and the chest (asthma).

Allergic rhinitis is a common condition that affects 10 to 15 percent of children and adults. Its most obvious form, commonly referred to as *hay fever*, occurs on a seasonal basis, usually in the spring and fall, in response to certain pollens. Symptoms typically include nasal congestion, nasal discharge, sneezing, and itching of the nose. Eye symptoms (*allergic conjunctivitis*), such as itching, redness, and tearing, frequently accompany this so-called seasonal allergic rhinitis.

A second type, called *perennial allergic rhinitis*, occurs year round in response to one or more indoor allergens such as dust mites and animal danders. Although less dramatic than the seasonal variety, this condition often leads to severe chronic nasal congestion. In addition, many people with perennial allergic rhinitis experience a worsening of their symptoms during the hay fever seasons. Both forms of allergic rhinitis are frequently complicated by secondary infections of the nose and sinuses.

Asthma occurs in 5 to 10 percent of Americans. In this condition, allergens and other triggering agents, such as infections, exercise, cold air, and cigarette smoke, cause muscle spasms, swelling, and excess mucus production in the air passages of the lung. These events lead to narrowing, or constriction, of these airways. The most common symptoms of asthma are coughing, wheezing, and difficulty breathing. In extreme cases, asthma can be life threatening. Depending on a person's age, specific allergies can be a major trigger for asthma in up to 90 percent of patients. It is important to note, however, that many asthmatics, particularly adults, have no evidence of allergy and that allergy is rarely the sole cause of asthma. Most asthmatics are affected by a variety of triggers in addition to allergies.

Other allergic conditions include *eczema*, which is also called *atopic dermatitis*, and allergic reactions to foods, insect venoms, and drugs. Each of these conditions involves true allergic reactions, with a specific allergen causing symptoms in a previously sensitized person. However, with the exception of some cases of eczema, these conditions do not involve inhalant allergens and will therefore not be particularly relevant to the information provided in this book. It should be noted, however, that many infants and young children with eczema will go on to develop allergic rhinitis and/or asthma. For that reason, it may be reasonable to consider some environmental control measures in an effort to prevent the development of these respiratory allergies. Allergy prevention will be discussed in detail in Chapter 20.

A host of other conditions have been incorrectly attributed to allergy. Some of them may involve symptoms that are typical of allergic disease and cause understandable confusion. For example, some people blame their nasal congestion on allergy when it is really the result of a chronic sinus infection. Other conditions, however, such as behavioral problems in children, bear no resemblance to the usual manifestations of allergy. Here we will speak of a condition as being allergic only if it meets the criteria we have mentioned, in which the body reacts to a foreign substance, after a period of exposure and sensitization, through specific mechanisms in the immune system.

CHAPTER 3

What Is an Allergen?

An allergen is any foreign substance that triggers the allergic process described in the last chapter. The word *allergen* therefore describes a wide range of substances, including foods, pollens, molds, animal danders, insect venoms, and medications. Most allergens are naturally occurring substances (for example, pollens, dust mites, animal danders, foods, and insect venoms), although a few are man made (for example, certain drugs). This diverse lot is tied together by the fact that they are all capable of prompting the body to produce specific IgE antibodies.

For the purposes of this book, we will focus primarily on airborne allergens, which are also called *aeroallergens.* Aeroallergens can be grouped in a variety of ways, but for the most part we will use two general categories: those that occur in outdoor environments and those that occur in indoor environments.

The most common outdoor allergens are the pollens of various trees, grasses, and weeds as well as certain types of mold. They generally enter the atmosphere during specific seasons and produce the typical symptoms of seasonal allergic rhinitis (hay fever). As will be described in more detail later, these seasons generally occur at very predictable times each year in any given geographical region.

Indoor allergens are usually present on a year-round (perennial) basis; most important among these are dust mites and animal danders, with cockroaches and certain mold species also being important in some areas. These allergens tend to produce chronic symptoms that are more persistent, but usually less obvious, than those of seasonal allergic rhinitis. In addition, both indoor and outdoor allergens are capable of inducing asthmatic reactions.

Aeroallergens share several important characteristics. For each allergen, one or more specific components are responsible for the induction of the IgE response and are referred to as *major allergens*. For example, although a grain of ragweed pollen is made up of many components, one specific subunit brings about most of the allergic reaction. Chemically, these major allergens are all proteins or glycoproteins (a protein plus a sugar). When airborne, they are carried on microscopic particles. Pollen grains are an example of one sort of airborne particle, whereas a flake of cat dander would be another. These airborne particles range in size from less than five microns (extremely small; one micron equals one millionth of a meter) to greater than sixty microns (larger but still only visible with a powerful microscope).

The capacity of any airborne allergen to cause an allergic reaction depends on two major factors. The first is a property called *allergenicity*, which refers to the ability of a substance to stimulate the production of specific IgE antibodies in susceptible individuals. A substance's allergenicity in turn depends on its size and its chemical structure. Some substances are ideally suited to interact with the immune system to initiate the process of sensitization, whereas others are virtually incapable of doing so. The highly specific nature of this process is best demonstrated by the fact that making minute changes in an allergen's chemical structure can dramatically reduce its allergenicity.

The second major determinant of an allergen's potential to cause disease is its concentration in the environment. This in turn relates to both its production (for example, the number of pollen grains which a ragweed plant produces) and its ability to become and remain airborne. Thus, the ideal allergen would be produced in high concentrations, would remain airborne for extended periods, and would stimulate a brisk IgE response.

I would like to focus for a moment on the factors that determine pollen levels in the outdoor air. First, each plant is genetically programmed to release its pollen at a specific time of year. However, in addition to these seasonal influences, it is well known that different plants release dramatically different amounts of pollen into the atmosphere. The most important factor underlying these differences relates to the means by which a plant's pollen is carried from one plant to another. Pollens carry a plant's genetic material so they must be transported to other plants of the same species for reproduction. This process is called *pollination*. They can be transported from one plant to another by one of two means: insects or air. The reason that some plants have developed bright, colorful, perfumed, nectar-containing flowers is to attract insects to pick up and carry their pollen. This process is very efficient such that these plants may only need to produce a few hundred pollen grains, whereas a plant that depends on the air for pollination may need to produce millions.

The pollens produced by plants with brightly colored flowers rarely cause allergy. They are generally not produced in sufficient numbers and, in addition, their pollen grains are large and are designed to stick to a plant's surface or to insects' feet rather than to become airborne. On the contrary, most of the plants that cause significant allergies use the air to transport their pollen. They produce far more pollen and are less attractive because they have no need to draw insects to themselves. It is interesting to note that the more colorful plants are often falsely accused of causing allergies because they happen to bloom at the same time of year that some of the more allergenic plants are pollinating. For example, so-called "rose fever" is caused not by rose pollen, but by pollen that is being released into the air by trees and grasses at the same time of year.

The concentration of a particular pollen in the atmosphere depends not only on the number of pollen grains that are produced, but also on the ability of that pollen to stay airborne once it is released. Smaller pollen grains tend to be more buoyant, remain airborne for longer periods of time, and disseminate more widely. Some pollens have also developed tiny air sacs that make them even more buoyant. These properties make for more effective pollination, but also increase the chance that a pollen will find its way into our noses and lungs. Larger pollens are less likely to trigger allergic reactions, and, in fact, some pollens (such as corn pollen) are so large that they fall rapidly to the ground when they are released and are virtually incapable of causing disease even though they may be released in high numbers.

The size of the pollen grain (or other particle) on which an airborne allergen travels is also important after it reaches us because it largely determines where it will be deposited in our respiratory tracts. Small particles are more likely to make it down into the bronchial passages of the lungs where they may cause asthmatic reactions, whereas larger particles are more likely to be trapped in the nose and induce an allergic reaction there.

As I will discuss in more detail in Chapter 6, there are several different means of identifying and measuring allergens. For outdoor allergens, pollen and mold spore counts have been the most popular for decades and are still the primary means used both to identify and measure these allergens. Counts are performed by exposing a collecting unit, usually a greased microscope slide, to outdoor air using one of several different sampling devices. These slides are then viewed under a microscope so that pollens and mold spores can be identified and counted. For indoor allergens, methods are now available to measure the levels of dust mite, cat, dog, mold, and cockroach allergens in house dust and air samples.

A great deal is known about both allergens and the allergic reactions that they cause. This information is extremely important in the design of environmental control measures. In subsequent chapters I will discuss the common allergens and their control in more detail. First, however, I will outline the diagnosis of allergy.

CHAPTER 4

How Is Allergy Diagnosed?

Before we can help a person suffering from what seems to be an allergic ailment, we must make an accurate diagnosis. This chapter describes some of the procedures that have proved reliable in diagnosing allergy, along with some other tests that are commonly used but which have not yet been shown to be effective.

Without a doubt, the patient's history is our most important diagnostic tool. It provides a wealth of information, and it should therefore be taken with great care and in considerable detail, ideally by a physician experienced in taking care of allergic patients. I would like to review some of the aspects of the history which might help your doctor to make a diagnosis regarding allergies and asthma.

First, your doctor must know what symptoms you have. Do you have nasal congestion, frequent sneezing, or a runny or itchy nose? What color is your nasal discharge? Do your eyes ever water or itch? Do you have a cough, wheezing, or shortness of breath? Are your symptoms more severe at certain times of the year (for example, in the spring or fall)? Can you identify any specific triggers for your symptoms (for example, dust or a pet)? What medications have you used, and how well did they work? Do you have a past history of asthma, allergies, eczema, drug allergies, or frequent sinus or ear infections? Is there a family history of allergy? Finally, your doctor will also want detailed information about your home and work (or school) environments. This information will be particularly helpful in identifying any particularly relevant triggers for your symptoms and in the eventual design of environmental control measures specific for your allergies.

The next step in the diagnostic process is the physical examination. For possible allergy, your doctor will be particularly interested in examining your nose, eyes, lungs, and skin. For example, if you have allergic rhinitis, the lining of your nose may be swollen and pale in color. You may also have a clear nasal discharge. On the other hand, if the lining of your nose appears very red or if you have a colored nasal discharge, the diagnosis might be infection rather than allergy. Allergic eyes typically appear red and irritated. Wheezing in the chest usually suggests a diagnosis of asthma. Examination of your skin might reveal hives or eczema. It is also important to remember, however, that the physical examination in allergy can be quite normal if your symptoms happen to be quiescent at the time of the exam. Thus, you could be suffering terribly one day and then have a normal examination a day or two later, which is why your personal history is so crucial.

In most cases, your history and physical examination will be sufficient for a general diagnosis of allergy or asthma. However, you may require additional specific laboratory tests to clarify the diagnosis. For example, I am commonly asked to see children who have chronic cough or nasal congestion and who have failed to respond to the usual allergy medications. I can use allergy tests to define the specific allergies that are causing the symptoms and to devise treatments specific for those allergies.

Laboratory tests for allergy can be divided into two general categories: screening tests and specific allergy tests. *Screening tests* are designed to help rule in or rule out a general diagnosis of allergy. They do not identify specific allergies. The most commonly used screening test for allergy is the total IgE level. As mentioned in Chapter 2, IgE antibodies are produced by allergic individuals in response to specific allergens. Some of these antibodies are present in the blood, and together they comprise the total IgE level, which is often elevated in people with allergies. Although the test can be very useful in certain situations, it is limited by a large number of both false positive and false negative results. For example, it turns out that about 20 percent of people with definite allergies will have a completely normal total IgE level (even though they have enough IgE antibody for certain allergens to cause significant symptoms). This is called a false negative result. Conversely, about 20 percent of non-allergic individuals will have an elevated total IgE level. This is called a false positive result. This may occur because IgE antibodies are produced by the body for reasons other than allergy, such as to fight against parasite infections. The routine use of IgE levels in the diagnosis of allergy is therefore of limited value.

Another screening test for allergy is called the *eosinophil count*. Also as mentioned in Chapter 2, eosinophils are a type of white blood cell which play a major role in allergic reactions. A rise in the total eosinophil count in the blood can therefore serve as a general marker of allergy. However, like total IgE levels, the value of the total eosinophil count is limited by the fact that there is a great deal of overlap in results between allergic and non-allergic individuals. A more useful type of eosinophil count can be obtained by counting the number of eosinophils in nasal secretions. This is done by drying and staining nasal secretions and examining them under a microscope. The presence of large numbers of eosinophils is a very useful indicator of allergy. Moreover, the test is inexpensive, painless, and produces quick results.

There is a great deal of interest in the development of new and improved screening tests for allergy. The best of those currently available is a test called the Phadiatope. This test measures IgE antibodies to a group of common allergens. As opposed to the RAST described below, which measures IgE antibodies to individual allergens, the Phadiatope measures the response to a group of allergens and then interprets the result as positive or negative for a general diagnosis of allergy. In our study of this test, it was about 90 percent accurate in identifying both allergic and non-allergic individuals. Many commercial laboratories now offer this test, and other new tests are on the horizon.

As opposed to these general tests for allergy, other tests can be used to identify specific allergic sensitivities. Most common among these are skin tests and RASTs.

Skin tests are an old standby for allergists but are not generally available from other types of physicians because their use and interpretation require special training that most physicians do not receive. In the allergist's hands, skin tests are the most accurate of all tests for allergy and can be used to test for a wide variety of allergens. They are inexpensive, and their results are available within minutes. The allergist can therefore test quickly for a group of common allergens and provide immediate feedback for you. Skin tests have one major limitation: many of the allergens that are available have not been adequately tested or purified.

Skin tests can be done by two general methods: by puncture or intradermally. To perform a puncture (or prick) skin test, the technician will place a drop of an allergen on your skin (usually the forearm, sometimes the back) and make a tiny puncture through the drop into the top layers of skin. There are many devices for performing these tests. In an intradermal test, the technician will actually inject a small amount of allergen into the top layers of skin, using a small syringe and needle, thus introducing considerably more allergen. Thus, someone who is highly allergic will test positively to a puncture test, whereas a less allergic person may test positively only to an intradermal test. Whenever skin tests are performed, control tests are required for comparison. A solution of histamine is used for the positive control test to make certain that your skin reacts normally; all tests would be falsely negative if you had recently taken an antihistamine. Similarly, a drop of salt water is used as a negative control test because some people have such sensitive skin that they will react just to the trauma of the puncture (and will appear to be allergic to everything).

The number of skin tests needed when testing you for allergy varies tremendously with your age and the purpose of the testing. For example, if the purpose of the testing is to determine whether you are allergic to milk or to the new family cat, only those specific tests would be needed, in addition to the positive and negative controls. For a more general screening for allergy, a total of fifteen to twenty-five of the most common indoor and outdoor allergens is commonly used. In some situations, such as when your physician is going to prescribe allergy shots, far more extensive testing is required, and in many cases both prick and intradermal tests for each allergen are required.

RAST stands for *radioallergosorbent test*. These tests have been in use for some twenty years and have been refined to a point where they are now quite accurate specific tests for allergy. Many variations of this test have now also been developed, with names like VAST, MAST, and FAST. In these tests, your level of specific IgE antibodies against specific allergens is measured in a blood sample. Early on, there was tremendous variation in RAST results from one laboratory to another, but now most are fairly consistent. The main advantage of RASTs over skin tests is that no special training is needed to conduct them. A tube of blood can be drawn and sent to a laboratory, so you do not need to seek out the expertise of an allergist.

The main drawback to RASTs is their cost. Whereas skin tests cost about three to four dollars per allergen, RASTs cost between ten and twenty dollars each. Thus, even a small general screening for allergy, which might include about fifteen tests, would be rather costly. RASTs may therefore be most useful to answer limited or specific questions, such as whether or not you are allergic to dust mites or cats. When a full array of tests is needed, having an allergist conduct skin tests would generally be more cost effective. In addition to the advantages of skin tests, the allergist also has the expertise to select appropriate allergens for testing, interpret the test results, and provide more knowledgeable recommendations for your treatment.

Other tests for allergy are used mainly for research purposes. For example, in my research we perform "challenge tests" by exposing subjects to cats and measuring their reaction. The diagnosis of allergies to animals can be particularly difficult because of the prejudices and emotions that are typically involved. Many people will deny the validity of a positive allergy test to a family pet. If this occurs, the next step might be to arrange a trial separation from the animal. However, as will be described later, simply removing the animal from the home for a few days or even weeks may not produce accurate results because it sometimes takes several months after the animal has been removed for the allergen levels to subside significantly. The better procedure would be for the patient to stay away from home for a few weeks to see if the symptoms are reduced.

Other types of challenge tests, in which you are exposed directly to an allergen, can be used in a variety of different ways, most often to assist in diagnosing food allergies. Skin tests and RASTs for foods can be very difficult to interpret, in that it is common for a patient to test positively to a food that can actually be eaten without difficulty. The only way to sort out these situations accurately is with a "food challenge test." In such a test, you are given gradually increasing amounts of the suspect food. These tests are often done in a "blinded" fashion, in which you eat either a placebo or the suspect food, prepared in such a way that it cannot be identified. The main drawbacks to these tests are that they are time consuming and potentially dangerous. Because some patients may have severe reactions, these tests should only be administered in a hospital or office setting that is equipped to treat them.

Finally, there are many other tests that are of questionable accuracy or unproven effectiveness for diagnosing allergy and are therefore not recommended. These include sublingual (under the tongue) drops, neutralization tests, injections of your own urine, cytotoxic tests, and a variety of other blood tests.

In summary, we have many tools at our disposal for the diagnosis of allergy. We paint the general picture using the history and physical exam. We can then employ screening tests, ideally in a limited way, to help clarify the diagnosis. Then, we can perform specific allergy tests to identify specific sensitivities. This final group includes RASTs, which will be most helpful for testing for a few specific allergens, and skin tests, which we will most often utilize to do more extensive evaluations for allergy. With this information, we will usually be effectively armed to treat all of your allergic problems.

CHAPTER 5

Common Allergens

As I discussed in Chapter 3, allergens are a diverse group of substances that are tied together by their particular ability to induce the production of specific IgE antibodies in susceptible individuals. Most allergens are naturally occurring substances produced by either plants or animals. Again, I will group them primarily by their occurrence in nature as either indoor or outdoor allergens. Common indoor allergens include dust mites, animal danders, cockroaches, and some molds. Common outdoor allergens include the pollens of various trees, grasses, and weeds and certain mold species. In this chapter I will examine these common allergens in some detail, and then in subsequent chapters I will describe specific environmental control measures for each of them.

DUST MITES

Dust mites are overall the most important of the indoor allergens. For decades, people have been diagnosed as being allergic to "house dust." We now know, however, that these people were not allergic to the house dust itself, but rather to specific components of house dust, such as animal danders, molds, cockroaches, and particularly, dust mites.

Dust mites are tiny (microscopic) eight-legged creatures that are closely related to ticks and spiders. They grow best where it is warm and humid, and they live predominantly on a diet of human skin scales. They have been found in high numbers in house dust samples from Europe, the United States, Central and South America, the Far East, and Australia. The only areas that appear to be relatively spared of dust mites are those with very dry climates or those at high altitude (greater than three thousand-meter elevation). It has also been postulated that the design of "tight," energy-efficient houses, with limited ventilation and higher indoor temperatures and humidity, has led to significant increases in mite levels over the past twenty to thirty years.

Two major dust mite species, named *Dermatophagoides farinae* and *Dermatophagoides pteronyssinus*, are the most important causes of dust mite allergy. Other species may also be important in more limited geographical regions. It has been shown that *D. farinae* is capable of surviving periods of lower humidity and therefore tends to predominate in climates that are less consistently humid. *D. pteronyssinus* is more likely to be the dominant mite in areas where humidity is consistently high. Seasonal variation in mite numbers may occur in some areas, with peaks occurring in the summer and fall. Mite-induced symptoms tend to be most prominent in the fall and early winter, however, when people spend more time indoors and seal their homes more tightly to conserve heat, which serves to reduce ventilation and increase mite exposure.

The most important dust mite allergen is actually a digestive protein found in their feces. Other mite allergens are found in body parts. The allergens are carried on relatively large particles, predominantly fecal pellets, which tend to settle rapidly after being disturbed.

Dust mites are not common components of surface dust but instead grow best in fabrics such as mattresses, pillows, bedding, carpets, upholstered furniture, and stuffed animals. Environmental control for mites must therefore focus on these prime areas. Your strategies for mite control should follow three general principles: 1) you can remove the sites of mite growth from your immediate environment; 2) you can place impermeable barriers between you and the mites; or 3) you can wash the mites out of some of the fabrics in which they reside. I will describe these methods in detail in Chapter 9.

ANIMAL ALLERGENS

Animal allergens are another extremely important cause of allergic disease. This is both because many animals produce potent allergens and because people insist on close contact with them. Currently, more than half of all the homes in the United States house at least one cat or dog, with a total pet population of more than one hundred million. In addition, cat and dog allergens are present to a small degree even in most homes that do not currently house an animal. This may occur either because a previous resident of the home owned a cat or dog or because the allergens were carried into these homes from another home where animals were present. Other important animal allergens come from guinea pigs, hamsters, rabbits, rats, and mice, which are also commonly kept as pets in the home as well as in schools and even pediatric hospitals. On farms, horses, cows, and other animals can also be important causes of allergic disease.

Several major animal allergens have now been identified and defined. These allergens are commonly found in secretions from cats and dogs and in the urine of most rodents. For example, *Fel d* I, the major allergen of the domestic cat, is produced in saliva and in sebaceous (oil) glands of the skin. In dogs, major allergens have been detected in saliva, dander, and possibly urine. Although an animal's hair may carry some allergen and serve as a visual marker of the animal's presence, the hair itself is not an allergen. The type or length of an animal's hair is therefore not important. Moreover, although we know that some animals produce far more allergen than others, the differences do not seem to be related either to specific breeds or to the length of the animal's hair. So, contrary to popular belief, there are overall no differences between long haired and short haired animals with regard to the amount of allergen that they produce, and there are no specific breeds of cat or dog which should be considered safe for allergic people.

It is presumed that the secretions containing these animal allergens dry on dander, fur, bedding, carpeting, and other objects and then become airborne when these objects are disturbed. Studies of airborne cat and rat allergens have shown that they are carried on particles that range in size from very small to very large. The small particles are particularly important because they have the potential to remain in the air for hours after they are disturbed.

Studies have also shown that cat allergen appears to be sticky and to adhere to walls, clothing, and other surfaces. The same is probably true of dog and other animal allergens. This property certainly contributes to that fact that these allergens are found even in homes that have never had pets. It should also be made clear, however, that allergen levels are far higher in homes that do contain pets and that the levels found in homes without pets are rarely high enough to cause disease.

Whenever possible, avoidance is obviously the best cure for animal allergy. When complete avoidance is not possible, however, there are other measures that will help to reduce exposure to animal allergens. I will describe these and other measures in detail in Chapter 10.

COCKROACHES

Cockroaches have also recently been recognized as a major source of indoor allergens, particularly in inner city areas. Major allergens from both the German and American cockroach have now been identified and characterized. Although the exact sources are not presently clear, these allergens may be contained in the insects' feces, body parts, and even saliva. In homes, cockroach allergens are widely distributed, with the highest allergen levels occurring in kitchens and other food storage areas.

Although cockroach allergy was not even recognized until the 1960s, we now view cockroaches as a major cause of allergic disease. Positive skin tests to cockroach allergen have been found in up to 50 percent of allergic patients in some areas, and in some cases cockroach sensitivity represents the sole cause of a patient's house dust allergy. Cockroach allergy may cause both asthma and allergic rhinitis.

Although a great deal is known about the control of cockroaches with regard to chemical extermination, no definitive studies have as yet been reported on the specific reduction of cockroach allergen in home environments. This may be a particularly difficult problem because of a variety of logistical problems, particularly in inner city dwellings. It is critical that effective programs for cockroach control be devised, however, and studies are in progress at the present time. Chapter 11 reports current control strategies.

MOLD ALLERGENS

Molds occur in both indoor and outdoor environments in many forms; we know them as molds, mildew, yeast, and fungi. Indoors, molds may grow wherever there is sufficient surface moisture and adequate temperature. Although there may be some seasonal variation in response to changes in temperature and humidity, these indoor molds commonly persist year round, particularly in warmer climates. Their favorite habitats are basement walls, window moldings, and bathroom walls and fixtures. You can also find them in food storage areas, garbage containers, decaying upholstery and foam rubber, household plants, and poorly maintained humidifiers, vaporizers, and air conditioners.

Outdoor molds favor fallen leaves, soil, thatch, moist debris, and damp surfaces. They become airborne, often in extraordinary numbers, when they are disturbed by lawn mowing, leaf raking, plowing, and other similar activities and therefore are particularly a problem in the summer and fall. According to some reports, mold spore counts peak in the afternoon. Levels of outdoor molds fall markedly with the onset of cold weather in the late fall or early winter. In Chapter 12 I will describe approaches to the control of both indoor and outdoor molds

Despite the vast variety of both indoor and outdoor molds, it seems that relatively few of them are common causes of allergic disease. Most important among these are *Alternaria* and *Cladosporium*, which are most prevalent in outdoor environments, and *Aspergillus* and *Penicillium*, which are most prevalent in indoor environments. The exact nature of most mold allergens still remains quite unclear in spite of extensive study. This fact has made the preparation of reliable mold extracts for diagnostic and therapeutic use difficult, with mold sensitivity remaining one of the more confusing areas in clinical allergy as well as a challenging area of research.

POLLENS

As I described in Chapter 3, pollens carry the plant's male genetic material and therefore act as fertilizing agents. Pollens are microscopic particles that are widely disseminated in outdoor air. In certain seasons, they may settle to produce a yellow dust on cars, railings, and other outside objects. Under the microscope, the pollen of each plant species is seen to have a distinct and characteristic appearance.

The major allergens for many pollens, particularly the grasses and ragweed, have been identified and characterized. Because the allergens from related plant species are often quite similar, it is common for people to become allergic to several plants from the same family. This is referred to as *cross-reactivity.*

Plants tend to shed their pollen in seasonal patterns. These so-called pollen seasons differ widely from region to region but are generally very predictable on a year-to-year basis in any given area. The accompanying figures provide a general outline of the pollen seasons in different areas of the United States. As you can see, tree pollens are generally the first to appear, arriving as early as January in the Southeast and later in the spring as one travels northward. Among the trees that most commonly cause allergy symptoms are oak, maple, Western red cedar, elm, birch, beech, ash, poplar, hickory, and cypress. Grass pollens then typically appear later in the spring and remain into the summer months. The most troublesome grass pollens are those of timothy, orchard grass, Bermuda grass, rye, sweet vernal, and certain blue grasses. Among the weeds, ragweed is by far the worst offender; its pollen appears in the late summer and early fall across much of the United States. Other weeds, which may pollinate from the late spring through the summer, include plantain, sage, pigweed, tumbleweed, and cocklebur. It is both interesting and fun to become familiar with the pollen seasons in your particular area. You can usually find pollen counts in your local newspaper and on TV, and following this information may help to explain exactly why your nose and eyes react the way they do at certain times of year.

Although pollens are located predominantly in the outdoor environment, substantial concentrations may also be present in house dust during the pollen seasons. As I will describe later, it is therefore very important to keep your doors and windows closed at those times of the year if you are pollen allergic.

It is clear that we are exposed to a phenomenal variety of allergens on a daily basis. No wonder so many of us have allergies!

PEAK POLLEN SEASONS

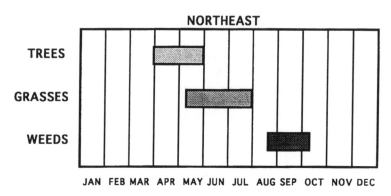

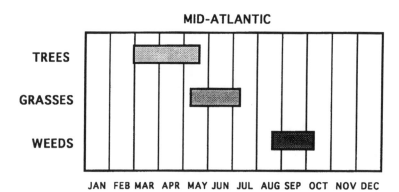

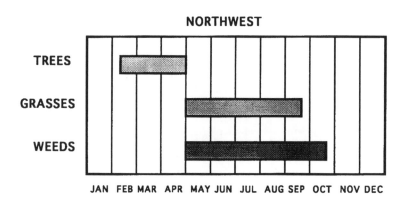

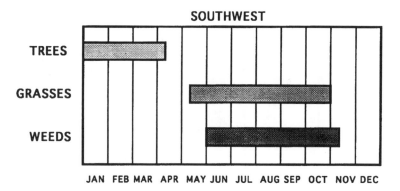

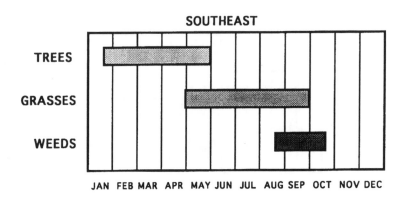

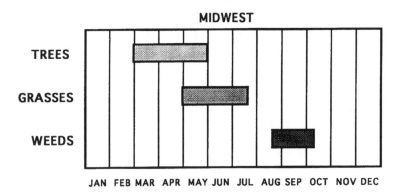

CHAPTER 6

Measuring Allergens in the Environment

I am sure that many of you have wondered what a pollen count really means. In this chapter I will describe pollen counts and other methods that are used to measure the allergens in the environment. I will also describe some new and very exciting techniques that can be used to measure indoor allergens such as dust mites, cockroaches, and animal danders.

For outdoor allergens, pollen and mold spore counts have been used for decades and are still the primary means of identifying and measuring these allergens. These counts are done by exposing a collecting unit, usually a greased slide, to outdoor air using one of several different sampling devices. The most common device is the rotating arm impactor (or Rotorod), pictured here. The device is set up either in an open area or on the roof of a one-story building. Clear plastic rods are attached to the arms of a rotating head. These rods are hidden except during specific

timed intervals, usually 10 minutes per hour, when the head ro-
tates, causing the rods to flip downward. Pollen grains and mold
spores that are floating by the sampler may then strike and stick
to the rods, which are then examined under a microscope. It is
remarkable to see just how many pollen grains and mold spores
can end up on these tiny rods!

Other devices that may be used to measure pollens and
molds are gravity samplers and suction filters. Gravity samplers
simply allow pollens and spores to settle onto greased slides.
Their advantage lies in their simplicity. However, they are less
accurate than rotating arm impactors because a lively wind can
blow the pollens right past the sampler. Suction samplers actually suck a specified amount of air through a filter. They are the
most accurate measuring devices, but they are rather cumbersome and expensive.

The slides from these devices are viewed under a microscope
so that the trapped pollens and spores can be identified and
counted. The pollens and spores of each different plant and mold
species have a distinctive appearance under the microscope. The
shapes of some of the more common pollens are shown in the
accompanying figure. Pollens are characterized not just by different shapes and sizes but by different markings on their surface.
Some of them, like the ragweed pictured here, have distinctive

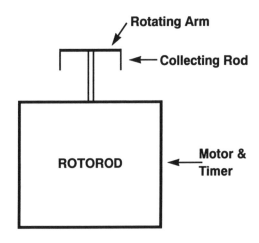

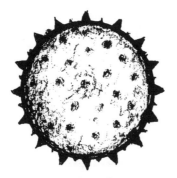

Ragweed

spikes on their surface. Others have characteristic holes, burrows, pockets, or other identifying marks.

Pollen counts and mold spore counts, though not perfect, do provide an excellent means of studying trends in outdoor allergen levels from one year to another. The annual rise and fall in specific pollen counts which were diagrammed in Chapter 5 are highly correlated with the symptoms of seasonal allergic rhinitis (hay fever) which so many people experience.

Over the last few years scientists have developed highly accurate laboratory tests that make it possible to measure the levels of the major indoor allergens in house dust samples collected from home environments. Tests are now available for measuring dust mite, cat, dog, mold, and cockroach allergens. Although the tests were originally developed for research purposes, several commercial laboratories now offer them for clinical use. For example, you could send a sample of dust to these laboratories and have it analyzed for the level of dust mite or cat allergen in your home. Although this information is not necessary for every patient with allergies, it can be very helpful in some situations to identify the specific triggers for a patient's symptoms or to monitor the effects of specific environmental control measures. Please ask your allergist if you would like further information on such tests.

Thus, we have tools to measure allergen exposure which range from the relatively simple to the high tech. This is an exciting area that will undoubtedly continue to provide new and useful information in the coming years.

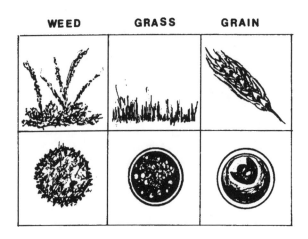

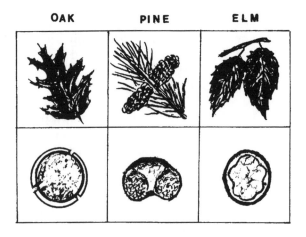

Common pollens

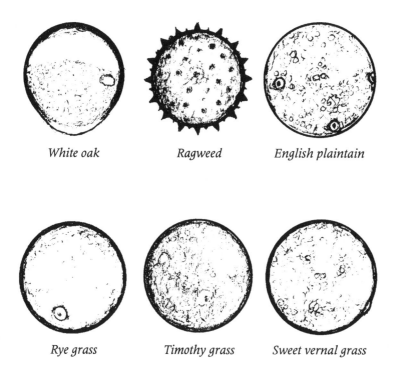

White oak   Ragweed   English plaintain

Rye grass   Timothy grass   Sweet vernal grass

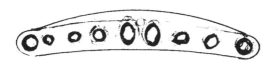

Helminthosporium
(a mold spore)

CHAPTER 7

Allergy Treatment Options

Before we move on to the specifics of environmental control, I would like to review each of the major treatment options that we have available for allergic rhinitis and asthma. These fall into three general categories: medications, allergy shots, and allergen avoidance.

MEDICATIONS FOR ALLERGIC RHINITIS

Most patients with allergic rhinitis have experimented with a variety of over-the-counter (OTC) medications before they decide to consult their doctor. These drugs are primarily antihistamines, decongestants, or a combination of the two. Antihistamines are designed to block the effects of histamine, one of the chemical mediators released by mast cells in allergic reactions, and they relieve sneezing, runny nose, and itching. Decongestants shrink swelling in the nose by constricting blood vessels and hence may help to relieve nasal congestion.

Examples of common antihistamines include OTC medications like Benadryl, Chlor-Trimeton, and Tavist and prescription medications such as Atarax (hydroxyzine), Seldane, Claritin, and Hismanal. Decongestants include Sudafed (OTC) and Entex (prescription). There are also decongestant nasal sprays such as Dristan and Neo-Synephrine. Combination products, which include both an antihistamine and a decongestant, are also very commonly used; examples of these include Dimetapp, Bromfed, Rynatan, and Seldane-D.

If you have mild allergic rhinitis, antihistamines and decongestants, even the OTC varieties, are generally effective. Their main drawback is their side effects. Antihistamines commonly cause drowsiness and lethargy, although in some people, especially children, they may have the opposite side effect and trigger hyperactivity. These side effects can be largely avoided with some of the newer prescription antihistamines, including Seldane, Claritin, and Hismanal. Unfortunately, these medications are more expensive and are currently only approved for adults and children over the age of twelve.

The most common side effects of decongestants are sleeplessness, shakiness, and hyperactivity. Although these side effects are mild in most people, they can be severe enough in some to limit their use, especially in young children. In adults, they may occasionally cause high blood pressure, increased heart rate, and bladder problems. The most significant side effects of these medications, however, are seen in people who overuse decongestant nasal sprays. After a few days of use, people commonly experience increased swelling of the lining of the nose as each dose wears off. This so-called rebound congestion can become so severe that some people only feel relief by using more of their spray, truly creating a sort of dependence. It is therefore recommended that these sprays not be used for more than two or three days at a time.

Unfortunately, some people fail to get adequate relief from even prescription antihistamines and decongestants. The reasons for this failure are obvious when you consider the nature of the allergic response as I described previously: these medications simply may not treat the severe swelling and inflammation that play such a large role in chronic allergic rhinitis. Even a perfect antihistamine would block the effects of only a single mediator—histamine—in what is actually a complex sequence of events involving many different mediators. Moreover, decongestants turn out to be fairly weak in their ability to reduce nasal swelling. They shrink the swollen tissue somewhat, but they do nothing to relieve the intense inflammation that underlies the swelling. Other medications may therefore be needed to control more severe cases of allergic rhinitis. These are all prescription medications that will require a trip to the doctor.

One such medication is called Nasalcrom (cromolyn sodium). Although just how it works is not entirely clear, it probably acts by inhibiting the release of mediators from mast cells, thereby blocking both the immediate and late components of the allergic response. It is extremely safe and has almost no side effects. However, it is only modestly effective in patients with severe allergic rhinitis, and it generally must be used four times a day, which is not an easy feat for most of us.

Another important group of medications for the treatment of allergic rhinitis is the steroid nasal sprays. Short of taking steroids by mouth, these are overall the most effective medications that are currently available. They are most capable of reducing the inflammation that causes the nasal swelling and congestion seen in people with severe allergic rhinitis. The currently available nasal steroids are beclomethasone (Vancenase and Beconase), triamcinolone (Nasacort), flunisolide (Nasalide), budesonide (Rhinocort), and dexamethasone (Decadron). Except for Decadron, these medications are broken down very quickly in the body after they are administered, which means that they can be given quite safely even though they are steroids. Their main side effects are irritation of the nose and occasional nose bleeds. However, these medications are indeed steroids, and you should use them with some caution, especially for children. They are best reserved for more severe cases and reduced to the smallest effective dose. For example, although at first you may need two sprays into each nostril twice a day to get relief, after a time you may maintain the same benefit with just one or two sprays in each nostril per day.

The strongest medications for the treatment of allergic rhinitis are steroids that can be taken by mouth, like prednisone, or given by injection. You should reserve these medications for the most severe cases and not use them for prolonged periods of time, unless absolutely necessary. If you require oral or injected steroids over an extended period you are at risk for developing serious side effects such as a slowing of growth (in children), bone thinning, muscle weakness, a round (moon-like) face, weight gain, cataracts, and suppression of the adrenal gland (which is needed to produce your body's natural cortisone and adrenaline). These side effects can be devastating, and you should make every attempt to avoid them.

MEDICATIONS FOR ASTHMA

There are also several different classes of medications available for the treatment of asthma. These include beta-agonists, theophylline, cromolyn sodium, nedocromil sodium, and steroids.

Beta-agonists include medicines like albuterol (Proventil and Ventolin), salmeterol (Serevent), metaproterenol (Alupent), terbutaline (Brethaire), and epinephrine. These medicines belong to a more general class called *bronchodilators* because they dilate constricted airways by relaxing the muscle spasms that occur in asthma. You can take them by inhaler, nebulizer (a sort of mist treatment), injection, pills, or syrups. They are extremely effective in relieving acute attacks of asthma and in preventing asthma symptoms from developing during exercise or other stressful activities. Their side effects include tremor (shakiness), rapid heart beat, high blood pressure, nervousness, sleeplessness, and hyperactivity, especially when the oral forms are given to young children. These medications are best used to relieve occasional symptoms, rather than as a regular day-to-day medication. If you have mild asthma and infrequent symptoms, one of these medications may be all that is needed. If you have more severe asthma or frequent symptoms, it is best to use one of the maintenance therapies described in the paragraphs below.

Theophylline is also a bronchodilator. Examples of theophylline products include Slo-bid and Theo-Dur. Though generally quite effective in the treatment of asthma, these drugs also have a variety of potential side effects. Theophylline is related to caffeine and has similar side effects, including head-ache, stomach ache, nervousness, sleeplessness, and hyperactivity, which again is most common in young children. In some children theophylline may even cause learning difficulties. Excessive doses of theophylline can lead to very severe side effects, including seizures and heart arrhythmias (abnormalities in the heart rate or rhythm). Fortunately, it is possible to measure blood theophylline levels to help guard against these dangerous side effects.

Cromolyn sodium, which is marketed for asthma as Intal, is available both as an inhaler and for nebulization. This is the same drug that is used in Nasalcrom to treat allergic rhinitis. It is extremely effective as a preventative medication for asthma. It has little or no effect if you are already wheezing, but rather it works to prevent the wheezing from occurring. It is particularly effective when you take it on a daily basis. Like cromolyn for the nose, Intal is also an extremely safe medication with very few side effects. Its main drawback is that it may not be potent enough to help you if you have severe asthma.

Nedocromil sodium is a relatively new preventative medication that is currently approved for use by adults and children over the age of twelve. When you use it on a daily basis, it is at least as effective as cromolyn sodium in preventing asthma symptoms. Aside from complaints about its taste, it is extremely safe with very few side effects.

Just as in allergic rhinitis, steroids are generally considered the most effective medications for asthma. Preparations similar to those used for allergic rhinitis are available as inhalers. They are marketed as Vanceril and Beclovent (beclomethasone), Azmacort (triamcinolone), and AeroBid (flunisolide). Steroids such as prednisone, which are taken by mouth, are also commonly used for asthma, particularly to control more severe attacks. As I have mentioned, however, these medications have a long list of potential side effects that we must strive to minimize or avoid altogether.

Although the medications described here comprise the vast majority of those used for the treatment of asthma, a variety of others may be used in select cases. For example, a medicine called Atrovent, which is a weak bronchodilator unrelated to those listed above, may have a role in some cases. And if you have very severe asthma, particularly if you suffer from the side effects of excessive steroid use, other treatments are available for use on an experimental basis.

All of the asthma medications I have described thus far are available only by prescription. There are, however, also a number of OTC preparations, such as Primatene Mist and Bronkaid tablets, both of which are types of bronchodilators. Most experts agree that for asthma you should minimize or avoid altogether the OTC medications. Asthma is a serious illness that needs to be carefully monitored by a physician.

Finally, you may have noticed that I have not mentioned antihistamines and decongestants as treatments for asthma. In fact, you will even see warnings on the labels of many such medicines saying that they should not be used by asthmatics. It turns out that they are safe for most people with asthma, although it is a good idea to check with your doctor before trying them. In addition, there is now even some encouraging research suggesting that some of the newer antihistamine preparations may have some role in asthma treatment.

ALLERGY SHOTS

Allergy shots, which are also referred to as *immunotherapy* or *allergy injection therapy*, have been used for decades to treat both allergic rhinitis and asthma. The general principle of allergy shots is quite simple: gradually increasing amounts of the allergens to which you are sensitive are injected over time in an effort to increase your resistance (tolerance) to those allergens. Your doctor will first perform allergy tests to determine the specific allergens that are causing your symptoms, and then he will prepare a weak solution of the offending allergens. You will receive gradually increasing doses of this solution, usually on a weekly basis, until you reach a full dose. You will then be given this dose, which is also called a *maintenance dose*, for years, usually once every two to three weeks. It usually takes four to six months to achieve a maintenance dose, and this dose contains one thousand to ten thousand times more allergen than the dose given in the first injection. The hope is that your nose and/or lungs will become that much more tolerant to the allergens contained in the shots.

For some patients allergy shots can be extremely helpful. They probably work best for patients with seasonal allergic rhinitis, in whom the vast majority have a significant reduction in their symptoms. While they work for most patients with perennial allergic rhinitis and asthma, their failure rate may be higher for those conditions. For patients with animal allergies, shots may not be effective enough to enable them to live with an animal to which they are highly allergic. Finally, allergy shots seem to worsen many cases of severe eczema, and they presently have no role in the treatment of food allergies.

Even if you clearly seem to benefit from immunotherapy, the shots always entail certain drawbacks and potential risks. Most importantly, each shot carries the risk of causing an allergic reaction, which could potentially be serious. The most common reactions are localized swelling at the site of the shot. This is expected to some degree, and small reactions can usually be ignored. The more serious reactions occur away from the site of the shot, such as the development of hives on other areas of the body. The most dangerous reactions include wheezing or even anaphylaxis, in which you may develop difficulty breathing, wheezing, swelling of the throat, or a dangerous drop in your blood pressure. These reactions can be fatal if they are not treated promptly. Most of them occur within the first thirty minutes after the shot is given, which is why you are asked to remain in the doctor's office for a period of time after receiving your shot.

The other major drawbacks to allergy shots are expense, inconvenience, and pain. The expense of allergy shots, which includes both the cost of the solutions and the cost of the injections, can be substantial if not covered by your insurance. A typical range would be $400 to $600 per year. In addition to the expense, allergy shots always involve some inconvenience. Going to your doctor's office every week and waiting around after each shot is hard for anyone. And for some people, especially young children, the fear of the injections makes this form of treatment a distinctly unpleasant experience.

In balance, although allergy shots are extremely helpful for many patients, it is generally recommended that they be reserved for select cases. They should generally be considered the last line of treatment for most people and should only be used after appropriate medications and environmental controls have failed. Active research on allergy shots is ongoing, and there is a chance that they will become more safe, effective, and convenient with time. Until that time, however, in view of the excellent results that most people achieve with other treatment, their risks and other drawbacks will outweigh their benefits for the majority of patients.

ALLERGEN AVOIDANCE

To many people, the practice of allergy has become virtually synonymous with the administration of allergy shots. This is very unfortunate because although allergists are certainly the best trained to prescribe allergy shots, it should not be their primary strength or function. Rather, the true strength of allergists lies in their ability to diagnose a patient's allergies specifically and then prescribe logical solutions for the avoidance of those allergens. Thus, allergen avoidance should be considered early in the management of all patients with significant allergic disease. It will complement the use of medication in most and even replace it in some. When that combination fails to provide adequate relief, allergy shots should be implemented as the last line of defense.

In the remainder of this book I will concentrate on methods of environmental control and allergen avoidance.

PART 3

Allergen Avoidance and Environmental Control

CHAPTER 8

A General Approach to Environmental Control

As you could no doubt gather from the conclusion to the last section, I believe that allergen avoidance should be part of the treatment plan for anyone with significant allergies. This form of treatment is not just the safest and most logical, it can also be the most effective. Some of the most dramatic results in allergy and asthma research support this notion, and in fact allergen avoidance can be the closest thing to a cure for many people.

In the following chapters I will outline environmental control techniques for common allergens. I will discuss each allergen separately because each needs to be viewed as a specific issue. Although there is some overlap in the methods that are used, for each allergen there are specific measures to employ for successful control. Moreover, the approach to each patient must be individualized on the basis of his or her specific allergies, the severity of the symptoms, and the details of the environment. Giving each patient the same prescription for environmental control would be just as inappropriate as giving them all the same medication or allergy shot.

For each allergen, I will therefore outline specific control measures. For most, I will advise a stepwise approach that will begin with some very simple steps for you to take. Then, if necessary, you can move on to more complicated or expensive procedures, which you should generally undertake only after testing has identified your specific allergies. For example, if you suspect that you are allergic to dust mites, you might take some simple, commonsense precautions just based on your suspicion. However, it could be an expensive mistake to remove all of the wall-to-wall carpeting from your home before a specific diagnosis of mite allergy has been made.

You should base your final decision regarding many environmental control measures on the severity of your symptoms. You might rightly choose not to remove a pet from your home if you are having only mild nasal symptoms, whereas you would be foolish not to do so if you were having severe, life-threatening asthma attacks secondary to an allergy to that pet.

In addition to allergens, many people also experience significant symptoms as a result of exposure to pollutants and other non-specific irritants in the environment. Cigarette smoke is the most important of these irritants, and its detrimental effects on the respiratory tract are well documented, even for those only exposed to secondhand smoke. And in addition to tobacco smoke, we are all exposed to a large and ever increasing array of pollutants both indoors and outdoors. I will therefore also address specific strategies for you to employ to reduce your exposure to these agents.

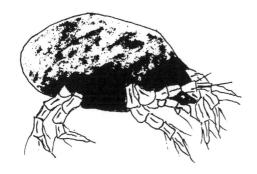

CHAPTER 9

Dust Mites

Dust mites are overall the most important indoor allergens. Doctors and patients alike had known for years that some people have allergic reactions upon exposure to dust, and from that came the general idea of "house dust allergy." We now know that people are not allergic to house dust in general but rather to certain specific components of the dust, among which dust mites are the most significant on a worldwide basis. We know that mites can trigger symptoms of asthma, allergic rhinitis, and even eczema. Recent research has shown that mite exposure may even be a cause of asthma in some patients—that is to say that some people with asthma may not have ever developed their disease had they not been exposed to high levels of mite allergen.

On the positive side, it has also been clearly shown that reducing exposure to mites can dramatically reduce symptoms in allergic individuals. This is even true in people with asthma. In fact, several studies have now demonstrated that mite avoidance can lead to dramatic improvements in asthma in both children and adults, sometimes to the point where they actually appear cured of their disease.

I described the ideal living conditions for dust mites in Chapter 5. I would like to review two major points from that section here because they are of critical importance to the design of dust mite control measures. First, dust mites live primarily in fabrics such as bedding, carpets, and upholstered furniture. They are not particularly common in surface dust—the kind of dust which accumulates on furniture and other objects. Second, dust mites thrive in warm, moist, humid environments. The only natural environments that significantly inhibit mite growth are those that are too dry, too cold, or too high (mites grow poorly at high elevations). Temperature is rarely a factor in indoor environments in this day and age, however. Even if a home is kept very cool, local environments like beds are usually warm enough to support mite growth.

There are three general strategies for the environmental control of dust mites. First, we can sometimes remove the objects in which they live and grow, such as carpets, upholstered furniture, and stuffed animals. Second, we can place physical barriers, such as plastic covers for mattresses and pillows, between them and us. And third, we can try to wash them out of some of the objects in which they reside. I will discuss these approaches in detail as well as several additional techniques that may be of use in some homes.

We should approach most environmental control in a stepwise fashion, and this is certainly true for dust mites. The first line of treatment should be relatively inexpensive and reasonable to consider for most people who suspect that they might be mite allergic. The second phase is more costly and should generally be reserved for those with proven mite sensitivity. The third level is yet more involved and should be limited to those with more severe disease. I make these distinctions because I have seen patients who were advised to take elaborate measures, costing thousands of dollars, and whose tests then showed that they were not allergic to mites after all. Although none of the measures was dangerous or harmful, they certainly were expensive.

Dust mite control usually begins in the bedroom. This is both because dust mites thrive in beds and bedding and because we spend many hours in direct contact with them there. Just think of the intimate contact that occurs between dust mites and our airways as we lie with our faces buried in a mite-contaminated pillow. If we can significantly reduce mite exposure for the 8 to 12 hours a day which are spent in the bedroom, we have an excellent chance of reducing symptoms.

In the bedroom begin mite control by placing impermeable plastic or vinyl covers on the pillow, mattress, and box spring. On bunk beds cover both mattresses, and do the same with any spare beds in the bedroom if at all possible. The plastic covers should encase these objects completely and be zippered securely. Simply covering the top of a mattress, as would be done for bed wetting, is not sufficient. The full covers can be purchased in most department stores or through the mail order suppliers listed in Chapter 19. Quality and cost vary considerably, mostly with regard to durability and comfort. Some of the more expensive covers are made with a layer of fabric which is much more comfortable than plain crinkly plastic. My usual recommendation is to buy the cheapest cover possible for the box spring and to consider more expensive covers for the pillow and mattress. Another option for the mattress is to use a mattress pad over the plastic encasement, as long as it can be laundered weekly in a hot cycle. The plastic covers themselves should be cleaned weekly with a damp cloth or sponge.

The next step is to remove all unnecessary fabric items, especially stuffed animals. Although washing them may help, I think that many stuffed animals remain contaminated no matter how often you clean them. I also believe that stuffed animals present a special risk because children often sleep with them pressed against their faces, creating the absolute maximum possible exposure.

Other items that you should remove from the bed include extra pillows, canopies, and comforters—especially down comforters. Replace them with items that can be laundered easily, and wash all bedding in a hot cycle at least once every two weeks. Just how hot the water needs to be has been a point of debate. It was originally stated that temperatures had to be above 160 degrees, a temperature that would impossible to achieve in most homes and which in any case would be extremely dangerous in homes with small children. A recent study, however, showed that a temperature of 130 degrees effectively killed 90 percent of the mites that were present. This temperature is still higher than safety experts would recommend for homes with small children, so you must exercise extreme caution. This study also showed that although lower temperatures did not kill mites, you could wash most of the mite allergen out of a fabric even in a cold cycle. Frequent washing at even low temperatures will therefore help to reduce mite allergen levels temporarily even if the mites are not killed.

Although dust mites certainly grow better in some pillows than others, it is important to note that no pillows are truly "non-allergenic" when it comes to dust mites. The issue of feathers and down is a particularly interesting one. We used to think that these substances were active allergens because so many people seemed to react to them. It turned out, however, that the real culprits were dust mites that grow magnificently in down. When I was growing up my allergist was therefore not entirely wrong when he said that I was allergic to feather pillows; the reasons were wrong, but the advice was perfect.

It has commonly been recommended that a water bed would be a safe alternative to a regular mattress encased in plastic. This seemed to make sense, and until recently I heartily endorsed the use of water beds. However, a 1992 report from Denmark said that mite levels on water beds were just as high as the levels on either spring or foam mattresses. Until there is convincing evidence to the contrary, I therefore now recommend that water beds not be used as a substitute for mattress covers.

A final option for reducing mites in mattresses involves using electric blankets. In one study, it was shown that you could reduce significantly the mite content of mattresses by running an electric blanket on a continuous basis. This presumably works by drying the mattress to a point at which mite growth is impaired. In spite of this information, however, I am very reluctant to recommend this because of a small but very real risk of starting a fire in the process of killing mites.

Although I have thus far emphasized the particular importance of mite control in the bed itself, you will not accomplish more complete avoidance unless you scrutinize carefully the rest of the bedroom. As I mentioned before, you should eliminate all fabric items if possible. Although I would certainly rather have stuffed animals on the dresser or a shelf than on the bed, it is best to remove them altogether. You should remove all upholstered furniture and replace fabric curtains. Some allergists urge that you remove books and other items that seem to collect dust. Although this certainly will do no harm, I am not convinced that these items are really a problem, as an accumulation of surface dust does not necessarily mean that mites are present. Carefully dusting once or twice a week should be adequate.

The next issue is carpeting. The first part is easy: get rid of all area rugs, except perhaps for a small one that you can launder easily. The next decision is far more difficult: what to do about wall-to-wall carpeting. This is a difficult issue because it can be quite expensive to have carpets taken up, particularly in newer homes, which usually do not have a usable floor underneath the carpet. Removing wall-to-wall carpeting will therefore also require installing a tile or wood floor in many homes. Because of the expense involved, you should probably take this step only after testing has confirmed the diagnosis of mite allergy. As I spoke to one family recently and informed them that there was no evidence of mite allergy in their child, they nearly cried as they told me they had just spent over $10,000 replacing all the carpets in their home upon the advice of their well meaning doctor.

I would therefore place carpet removal in the second tier of mite control measures. The problem with this advice is that it may not be possible truly to reduce mite exposure as long as there is a contaminated carpet in the bedroom. So, although I commonly begin with the control measures in the bed as described above, I encourage all patients with documented mite allergy to remove bedroom carpeting if at all possible. Once you have removed a carpet, you should damp mop or dust the floor weekly.

More frequent vacuuming is often suggested as an alternative to removing the carpeting. That solution is never as effective as carpet removal, however, because dust mites and their feces become so embedded in carpets that vacuum cleaners may not be capable of reducing their levels significantly. Some manufacturers claim that their vacuum cleaners are effective in removing mites from carpeting, but studies have actually shown that the concentration of mite allergen in a carpet is unaffected by vacuuming—that is, the reservoir of mite allergen in most carpets is so large that the concentration of allergen in the dust that is removed does not change with even prolonged vacuuming. In the end, however, because all of the dust that is removed does indeed contain mite allergen, the total mite burden in a carpet has to be reduced to some degree with frequent vacuuming. For that reason, it still makes sense to vacuum frequently (at least twice a week) if carpeting cannot be removed.

You need to be cautious while vacuuming because the vacuuming itself can blow tremendous amounts of allergen into the air. As I will describe in Chapter 19, this is actually the most important difference among vacuum cleaners. Some vacuum cleaners do a much better job than others of containing the allergen they pick up, whereas others expel high concentrations of allergen into the air (and into the vacuumer's face). The best solution is either to get a vacuum with an effective filtration system or to leave the vacuuming to someone who is not allergic to dust mites. People who are allergic should wear a mask if they have to vacuum and should air out the room thoroughly once the vacuuming has been completed. The only good thing about dust mites is that their allergen is carried on relatively large particles that settle quickly after being disturbed, so even if a room cannot be aired out, most of the mite allergen will have settled from the air within thirty minutes after vacuuming. Unfortunately, it will end up back in the carpet that we were trying to rid of mite allergen in the first place!

I just mentioned that airing out a room can be helpful. This is an important concept for all indoor allergens. One of the reasons for the increased incidence of mite allergy in recent years, along with the increased use of wall-to-wall carpeting, has been the trend toward tighter, more energy-efficient houses with less ventilation. Such houses tend to have higher indoor humidity levels and allow for less allergen removal by simple ventilation. The corollary to this concept is that anything we can do to increase ventilation may have a positive effect on indoor allergen levels, including dust mites. If you open a window even a crack you will significantly increase the ventilation in a room and help to reduce airborne allergen levels. Before getting too excited though, I will warn you that in a later chapter I will advise you to close windows in an effort to prevent pollens from entering the house. The best strategy will therefore depend on the season of the year and the patient's specific allergies.

The next issues in our battle to control dust mites are related to their reliance on moisture for growth. Mites grow best when the relative humidity is above 55 percent and grow poorly when it is consistently below 45 percent. Moreover, mite growth and mite allergen (feces) production increase substantially as the relative humidity increases above 55 percent. So anything that we can do to reduce humidity will help in our efforts to reduce mite exposure. Part of this problem is completely out of our hands: we can do nothing to control the general level of outdoor humidity in a given geographical area. Part of the problem, however, is entirely within our control and easily eliminated. I commonly see children who live with a humidifier or vaporizer running in their bedroom on a regular basis. In fact, one of the most common recommendations that pediatricians make for children with nasal congestion is to run a humidifier while they are sleeping. Although that may indeed help to ease the child's congestion, it may also encourage mite growth and in the end have a very negative effect. The wisest course is to ban humidifiers entirely from the rooms of children who have mite allergy. Central humidifiers in heating systems are also very prevalent. They are probably a lot less dangerous because they are usually only used during the drier parts of the year and, in any case, do not have as great an impact on humidity. Their use should still be limited, however, and people who are planning to install one should consider getting a humidity gauge for their home to make sure that humidity levels are not excessive. Ideally, indoor relative humidity should be kept at about 40 percent, a level that should be reasonably comfortable without encouraging mite growth.

Beyond limiting the use of humidifiers, there are three other important recommendations regarding the control of indoor humidity. First, air conditioners are extremely helpful and should be used in the warmer months of the year if at all possible. Second, a dehumidifier can be invaluable if your home is excessively damp, particularly in the basement and during the summer months. The final issue is critically important but often overlooked. It regards the use of carpets, especially wall-to-wall carpeting, over the cement floor of a basement. Because these carpets tend to be continuously moist, they pose a major health hazard for anyone with mite (or mold) allergy. A leading expert in this field, Dr. Thomas Platts-Mills at the University of Virginia, has even suggested that basement carpets be formally outlawed. They create some risk even when the basement is seldom used and are particularly dangerous when the basement is used as a family room, play area, or, worst of all, as a bedroom for a mite-allergic person.

The next steps for mite avoidance for the patient with significant mite allergy involve implementing some of the strategies that we have described for the bedroom in other areas of the home. It is reasonable to focus on one or two other rooms where you spend significant amounts of time. For example, in the family room or television room you could remove the carpeting and any replaceable upholstered furniture. I find that many children like to watch television lying on the floor with their face in the carpet. If you cannot remove the carpeting, it would be a great help to have the child sit off the floor on a non-upholstered chair. An inexpensive vinyl "bean bag" chair or a rocking chair can be a real hit that accomplishes both goals. And again, be particularly careful with basements.

The final steps for controlling mite exposure are primarily for those people with more severe symptoms. The first of these steps, however, involves something that many people have purchased long before ever coming to the allergist for evaluation. I am referring to air cleaners. These come both as small, portable room units and as central units that are installed in the home's heating or cooling system. I will discuss their use and function in more detail in Chapter 19, but here I would like to focus on their role in the control of dust mites.

I have already mentioned that dust mite allergens are carried on relatively large particles that remain airborne for only a few minutes after being disturbed. So if you went into a bedroom, only a tiny fraction of the total mite allergen would be airborne at any given time. The vast majority of the allergen would instead be in the bed, carpeting, and furniture. Since only the airborne allergen is available for removal by an air cleaner, there is little chance that even the most efficient unit could significantly reduce mite exposure, aside from immediately after disturbance (in which case the allergen settles quite rapidly anyway). I view dust mite exposure as occurring much more in local environments, such as the intense, intermittent exposure that occurs when you lie down in bed or turn your head in a contaminated pillow. These exposures will not be significantly affected by an air cleaner. If you are a mite-allergic patient who has not already purchased an air cleaner, I would therefore advise that you spend your money on more useful interventions first, such as mattress and pillow covers and carpet removal.

Another common question is whether it is helpful to have someone clean the heating ducts in your home. The concern is that these ducts may contain dust that will be blown through the house whenever the heat or air conditioning goes on. No one has investigated this question carefully, and it is not even clear whether or not this dust contains significant amounts of dust mite or other allergen. In addition, it also seems that the contractors that provide this service are quite variable—some do nothing more than run a long vacuum hose down into the ducts, whereas others break down the system and do a more thorough cleaning. A simple alternative to duct cleaning is to buy filters that fit over the vents into a room to help intercept any allergen that might be present in the incoming air.

A final strategy for reducing exposure to mites involves using certain chemicals designed to lower the mite allergen levels in carpets. There are two such products available for use at the present time (see also Chapter 19). The first is a solution of tannic acid. This chemical, used for many years in the tanning industry, has been shown to break down (denature, degrade) existing mite allergen. You buy it in a spray bottle and apply it directly to the carpet. Since this chemical has no effect on the mites themselves, you need to apply it at regular intervals to deal with the continued deposition of mite allergens. Although tannic acid has been on the market for several years now, a relatively small amount of information is available regarding its effectiveness. My assessment is that it does clearly help to reduce mite levels but that it will never be a replacement for carpet removal. It is best used as an adjunct to the methods described above in patients with significant mite allergy, particularly if there is a bedroom carpet that cannot be removed. Please be aware that products like this, unlike medications, do not need to undergo any testing for effectiveness before they are marketed.

The second product is benzyl benzoate, the first acaricide (dust mite pesticide) to be sold in the United States. This is another common chemical that has been used in a variety of industries. It is sold as a moist powder that is applied to a carpet, left to sit for several hours, and then vacuumed up. This product does kill dust mites. The problems, though, are how to get the existing mite allergen out of the carpet and how to keep the mites from reappearing as the chemical wears off. The first of these—getting the allergen out of the carpet—is the hardest to accomplish and may limit this product's ultimate success. You can overcome the second problem by repeating the application at regular intervals, although the ideal schedule is still not entirely clear. This product is also best reserved for people with significant mite allergy who are unable to remove their bedroom carpet.

Researchers are conducting experiments with these and several other new products, as well as with combinations of tannic acid and benzyl benzoate. We can reasonably hope that products such as these will have a much wider role in the treatment of mite allergy in the future. It certainly would be nice simply to kill the mites and not have to worry about all of these other steps. The major problem has been to identify chemicals that kill mites effectively but which are also safe for use in our homes. Although the two products above are safe and certainly will help some patients, they should be used in addition to, rather than instead of, the other measures I have outlined. You should consider them primarily for use in bedrooms where you cannot remove the carpet. The final point to consider is that these products are not inexpensive and that by the time you have gone through the repeated applications that will be necessary, you could have practically paid for carpet removal!

That closes our discussion of dust mite control. I have tried to present the information in a logical and stepwise fashion. Please now approach it that way. There is no need to do everything this weekend. Begin with the first line measures and proceed from there. The following summary should help to guide you further in your efforts.

ENVIRONMENTAL CONTROL FOR DUST MITES

First line measures:

- cover mattresses and pillows
- remove stuffed animals

- remove upholstered furniture and fabric-covered items from the bedroom
- control dust
- vacuum frequently
- improve ventilation
- stop using humidifiers
- place filters over heating vents

Second line measures:

- remove carpets, particularly in the bedroom and basement
- dehumidify

Third line measures:

- use air cleaners
- clean heating ducts
- use products that kill mites and destroy mite allergens

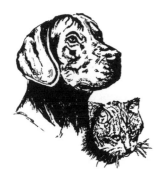

CHAPTER 10

Animal Allergens

Animal allergens are extremely important causes of allergic disease. Allergy to cats and dogs is most common, but virtually any furred animal can be a cause of allergy. For example, it is not uncommon for allergists to see patients with significant allergies to rodents, including rats, mice, gerbils, hamsters, rabbits, and guinea pigs, and farm animals, such as horses and cows. And among people working with more exotic animals, such as veterinarians, laboratory personnel, and animal caretakers, allergic reactions are even seen to less common animals, such as monkeys and the big cats. It is important to note that animals without fur, such as birds and fish, rarely cause inhalant allergies.

As I mentioned in Chapter 5, most of the common animal allergens are contained in either saliva, urine, or secretions from glands in the skin. The allergen may stick to the animal's hair, but, aside from that, hair has very little to do with an animal's allergen production. And although there can be substantial differences in allergen production among different animals, this has nothing to do with the amount or length of the animal's hair. The concept that a short haired dog or cat is less allergenic than a long haired animal is therefore completely erroneous. Also contrary to popular belief, there are no predictable differences in allergen production among the different breeds of dogs or cats, and there are definitely no breeds that should be considered safe for allergic individuals. So you need to be very careful of claims that you may hear that this or that breed that will not cause allergies in you or a loved one.

Animals are important causes of allergic disease for two main reasons. First, they produce remarkably potent allergens— proteins that lead readily to sensitization and subsequently to disease. Some animals, such as cats, are much better at this than others, with cat allergen being among the most potent of all allergens. The second reason is that we insist on having such close contact with animals. It is currently estimated that more than half of the homes in the United States house at least one pet, with a total pet population of over one hundred million! Cats have recently come to outnumber dogs as the most common household pet, and it is likely that this trend will continue. Cats are well suited to urban environments and require less day-to day care than dogs—a quality that is highly desirable with today's busy lifestyles.

It is estimated that between 5 and 10 percent of the people in the United States—that is, between 10 and 25 million Americans—are allergic to one or more type of animal. Among people who have other allergies, between 20 and 50 percent are also allergic to animals. And it turns out that because cats produce such potent allergens, allergy to them is about twice as common as allergy to dogs.

Allergic reactions to animals range from dramatic symptoms that occur within minutes of exposure to chronic, low grade symptoms that occur frequently in people who are living with an animal to which they are sensitive. Animal allergens often trigger both asthma and allergic rhinitis and are the most likely indoor allergens to produce eye irritation. I think that these eye symptoms are particularly common because people often go from petting an animal to rubbing their eyes, either inadvertently or because their eyes have begun to itch, thereby introducing a large dose of allergen to a very sensitive area. It is not uncommon to see severe eye swelling, particularly after exposure to cats.

This situation is obviously an enormous medical problem. In the remainder of this chapter I will review the steps that you can take to reduce your exposure to the animals to which you might be allergic. Please recognize that issues concerning pets are often emotionally charged, and in many instances you may need to have an allergy confirmed by testing before taking significant steps to reduce pet exposure. I have actually seen a marriage break up over a decision to remove a dog from a home, even after we had diagnosed a significant dog allergy in a child who had had repeated hospitalizations for asthma. On the other hand, I have seen children devastated by the removal of a family pet only to have it turn out that the pet was not causing any of their problems in the first place.

ENVIRONMENTAL CONTROL FOR ANIMAL ALLERGENS

As with dust mites, it is reasonable to approach environmental control for animal allergens in a stepwise fashion. Individualized treatment will depend primarily on the level of disease. If you have severe symptoms you will need to take more definitive steps than people with mild disease to get adequate relief.

From a strictly medical standpoint, it is relatively easy to argue that the most logical solution for someone who has an allergy to a pet is to take the animal out of the home. However, since pets play such an important role in many people's lives, it is reasonable to consider some alternatives to complete pet removal.

For patients with severe disease, it is usually necessary and appropriate to find another home for the pet, especially when the animal is causing asthma, a disease that can severely impair the quality of life and even be life threatening. As much as I like and appreciate pets, I take a very hard stand on this issue. In fact, I go so far as to consider as a form of child abuse a parent's refusal to remove a pet from the home of a child who has severe asthma related to an allergy to that pet. That may seem unfair, but some of these cases are more extreme than you could probably even imagine. For example, I saw one child who had been hospitalized for asthma more than seventy times and had nearly died on at least two occasions. Like his previous doctors, we felt that a major cause of the child's asthma was a severe allergy to the family's three cats. His parents had been told for years that the cats had to be removed from the home, but they had steadfastly refused to do so. You can imagine that we had a very frank discussion about these issues.

Once you have removed a pet, you must clean the house thoroughly to reduce the residual allergen content as rapidly as possible. We have found that it will typically take four to six months after a cat is removed for allergen levels to fall to a level that should no longer cause symptoms. Therefore, do not expect immediate relief. Similar studies have not yet been done for dogs, but the results would probably be similar. We find that these animal allergens are very "sticky" and therefore surprisingly difficult to remove.

You can accelerate the process of allergen removal by removing the major reservoirs of allergen from your home. As with dust mites, most important among these are carpeting and upholstered furniture. If removal is not possible, the allergen can be cleaned out of these objects gradually, although that is a very slow process. Neither frequent vacuuming nor even steam cleaning appears to speed the process of allergen removal significantly. Other steps that help to reduce allergen levels more quickly include increasing ventilation (by opening windows and air intake vents) and washing walls and other surfaces. This washing is important because cat allergen can be found adhering to walls and other surfaces in prodigious quantities. Finally, although it has never been studied, there is reason to suspect that heating ducts can become highly contaminated with animal allergens, so it might be helpful either to have them cleaned or to put filters over the vents.

The most reasonable approach for most homes is to pick the one or two rooms that the allergic person uses most often and to tackle those most aggressively. For example, it would once again make sense to work hardest on the bedroom to reduce exposure for the eight to twelve hours that a person would typically spend there each day. Simply removing the carpeting and upholstered furniture from the bedroom could make a tremendous difference very quickly. And since it has been shown that animal allergens may also remain in mattresses and bedding for extended periods, you should encase the mattress and pillows in plastic covers at the very outset. After you have dealt with the bedroom, your next target might be the family room or television room, where most people might spend another several hours per day.

We have studied some homes in which allergen levels remained persistently elevated even after the removal of a pet followed by vigorous cleaning. In one home, cat allergen levels remained essentially unchanged a full year after the cat had gone and, not surprisingly, the poor patient was still suffering miserably. In fact, she was doubly upset because she had lost her pet but not her symptoms! We were puzzled because she seemed to be a meticulous housekeeper but, after more careful investigation, we found that one room in the basement had never been cleaned adequately. The room served as a workspace for her husband who had spent countless hours there working on his hobbies with the cat lying at his feet. This room had an extraordinarily high allergen level a full year after the cat had been removed from the home. Unfortunately, this room was located next to the intake duct for the furnace, and the allergen was being blown out into the house every time the furnace went on. This case demonstrates that the cleaning process must be taken very seriously and that some detective work may be necessary to identify hidden pockets of allergen. Sometimes things are just not as simple as they seem.

One alternative to finding a new home for a pet is to keep the animal entirely outside. This is obviously better suited to some animals than to others, and it may only be possible to do safely in certain climates. In addition to these limitations, I have three general concerns with this approach. First, if the allergic person spends any amount of time with the animal outdoors, there may still be enough exposure to cause significant symptoms. Second, I worry that soft hearts will too often prevail in the event of rain or cold weather so that the animal will be brought indoors. And third, we must also always consider the pet's needs and quality of life. Quite simply, most pets would probably be safer, more comfortable, and happier living indoors in a new home.

For people with less severe allergies, a sufficient degree of avoidance may be possible without completely removing the offending pets from the home. The first step in this plan involves keeping the animals outdoors whenever possible and then restricting their movement within the home. In general, the more limited the mobility the better. Pets are best confined to areas without carpeting, such as the kitchen. Most importantly, the pet must be denied all access to the bedroom of the allergic person. And since allergen can travel within a home even when the pet cannot, the bedroom door should be kept closed at all times.

Removing the carpeting and upholstered furniture will also help to reduce allergen exposure when an animal is kept in the home. Although this should ideally be done throughout the house, it is again most important to concentrate on the bedroom and then possibly the family room. These fabrics continuously collect allergen, which is then released with vacuuming and other forms of disturbance. It is extremely difficult to clean the allergens out of these objects effectively, whereas damp mopping a wood or tile floor effectively removes allergen, as does wiping down non-upholstered furniture.

Increasing ventilation will also help to reduce exposure to animal allergens. An open window can be a tremendous benefit. In addition, as opposed to my comments regarding dust mite allergen, air cleaners may have a greater effect in the control of animal allergens. Because animal allergens tend to be carried on smaller particles than mite allergens, they typically remain airborne for longer periods of time after they have been disturbed. While airborne, these allergens are available for filtration, and an efficient air cleaner could remove them. As I will discuss in more detail in Chapter 19, either central or room units can do the job. My usual recommendation, however, is again to tackle the bedroom first with a room air cleaner. It is likely that this combination of restricting the animal from the bedroom, keeping the bedroom door closed, removing carpeting, encasing mattresses and pillows, and running an air cleaner will provide significant relief for many people with less severe allergies.

Two studies have shown that bathing the cat frequently helps to reduce the amount of allergen it sheds. Although both of these reports looked quite convincing, a third study published recently reported no benefit from cat washing. It makes sense that bathing could work by removing dander, sebaceous secretions, and saliva from a cat's coat. The positive studies found that a weekly bath using plain water is effective. Although it has not yet been studied, it may turn out that simply wiping the animal down with a wet rag will also help to reduce allergen levels. It certainly would be easier than trying to give most cats a bath! Although there have been no similar studies for dogs, it seems likely that regular bathing could eliminate much of the allergen from their coats as well.

You may have also seen products advertised as reducing allergen shedding when applied to an animal's coat. The best study that has been published to date found that one such product had no effect on allergen shedding from cats. My best guess at the present time is that they may work in the same way as cat washing, but they are unlikely to work any better than plain water.

The final step is to limit certain activities, including those directly related to the pet, especially brushing and grooming, as well as general cleaning practices. Leave all grooming chores to someone without allergies, if at all possible, and do all grooming outdoors. As with dust mites, cleaning, especially vacuuming with a standard vacuum cleaner, can stir up tremendous amounts of allergen, and someone with allergies should not do this without wearing a mask. Moreover, vacuuming is potentially more hazardous with regard to animal allergens in that the allergens are more likely to remain airborne for extended periods after disturbance. It is therefore a good idea to open a window while you are vacuuming to help clear the air as quickly as possible.

The best strategy for a person with an allergy to rodents can follow one of two general paths. First, if the rodents are unwanted, such as the home with rat or mouse infestation, undertake aggressive extermination. Follow the extermination with thorough cleaning and steps to block the rodents from reentering your home. This is particularly important in multiple dwelling units, in which it is best to have the extermination done in adjoining homes or apartments as well.

If a rodent is in your home as a pet, you will need different approaches. If you have severe symptoms, you probably should find a new home for your pet. If your symptoms are mild, it may be possible to keep the pet as long as you take certain precautions. You must keep the pet out of the bedroom and ideally out of the family room as well. Avoid or severely limit direct contact with the pet. If you have direct contact, wash your hands thoroughly so that allergen will not be rubbed into your eyes. Finally, it is very important to remember that cage cleaning is the activity most likely to stir up rodent allergens. Because most rodent allergens are contained in the urine, the bedding in the cage is typically saturated with allergen. Therefore no one who is allergic to rodents should do the cage cleaning without wearing a mask.

In summary, keeping pets out of your home is clearly the best way to deal with a significant animal allergy. If that is not possible, however, use the following strategies to help reduce your exposure to animal allergens.

- keep the pet outside as much as possible
- restrict the pet to the kitchen or other non-carpeted areas
- keep the pet out of the bedroom
- remove carpeting and upholstered furniture, especially in the bedroom
- keep the bedroom door closed
- provide good ventilation
- use an air cleaner
- wash the pet regularly
- avoid certain activities such as brushing and grooming the pet
- be careful with cleaning, especially vacuuming

If you observe all these strategies, you may be able to live with your pets in reasonable comfort. I will stress again, however, that if you have more severe allergies nothing short of complete avoidance will be sufficient, and anything less may be very hazardous to your health.

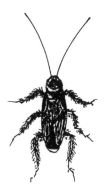

CHAPTER 11

Cockroaches

Over the last twenty to thirty years it has become apparent that allergy to the common cockroach is extremely widespread. Cockroaches were first recognized as a source of potent allergens in the 1960s when a study from New York City reported that nearly 40 percent of patients with asthma were allergic to cockroaches. We have now come to realize that cockroaches probably follow only dust mites and animal danders in their importance as indoor allergens and that in some settings they may be the most common and important indoor allergen of all.

Cockroaches are widely distributed around the world. In the United States, they are most common in urban areas. Even Northern cities have substantial cockroach infestation, and, as one travels further south, they become more and more prevalent, even in non-urban areas. The exact source of cockroach allergens is still not clear, but current research suggests that they may be contained in body parts, feces, and/or other cockroach secretions. The cockroach extracts that are currently used for allergy testing and immunotherapy are made from whole cockroach bodies.

Since the initial reports of cockroach allergy, cockroaches have been documented extensively as a major trigger of asthma. Although there has been less formal study on the subject, they also appear to be a common cause of allergic rhinitis. In fact, I have seen several patients with severe perennial allergic rhinitis who are sensitive only to cockroach. Effective environmental control is obviously an urgent need for many patients. The problem that we face, however, is that controlling cockroaches and their allergens in some homes may be an extremely difficult task. Although there has been extensive research on the control of cockroaches from an extermination standpoint, there is still very little information on the effects of extermination and other environmental control measures on cockroach allergen levels in home environments.

As opposed to many other allergens, most people are not even aware that cockroaches can cause allergy. Moreover, even those who are aware may be reluctant to believe that cockroaches are causing their symptoms. I have yet to have a patient come in and tell me that they have come to be cured of their cockroach allergy. For those who are aware of cockroach allergy, this may be the result of an unwillingness to admit that they have significant cockroach exposure or possibly a degree of disgust with the whole idea. The part of the history related to cockroach exposure always seems to make most people at least a little uncomfortable. It is certainly not pleasant to think that the reason your nose is so congested is that you are inhaling cockroach allergen on a regular basis. The bottom line is that testing is usually needed before a patient will truly entertain the idea of cockroach allergy.

Once a diagnosis of cockroach allergy has been made, the next step is to establish the degree of exposure in the patient's home or workplace. How often are cockroaches seen? What types of extermination have been tried? And possibly most important, in what type of dwelling does the patient live? Tackling a multiple-unit dwelling will be much more difficult than a single-family home.

As with all allergens, environmental control for cockroaches involves a logical series of steps. The first is aggressive extermination, which you can accomplish either through a professional service or independently using a variety of available products. A combination of sprays, bait traps, and boric acid can be very effective. Spray typical cockroach pathways, such as around kitchen cabinets and drawers, regularly with a chemical pesticide, such as chlorpyrifos (Dursban) or diazinon. Pesticide "bombs," which contain similar products, are also available for more widespread action. Boric acid powder is highly effective in killing cockroaches, and it can be sprinkled or blown under stoves, refrigerators, and other areas where cockroaches commonly hide. Be careful, though, that these products only be used in areas where children and pets will not come into contact with them. Finally, bait stations containing chemicals like hydramethylnon have been shown to reduce cockroach infestation for up to three months. If you live in an apartment building or other multiple-unit dwelling, it is critical that all of the units be treated so that the cockroaches cannot just go hide next door until the pesticides wear off.

After you have exterminated the cockroaches, the next step is to clean your home thoroughly to rid it of dead roaches and their debris. This is very important because without adequate cleaning it is entirely possible that cockroach allergen levels could actually rise as the dead bugs decompose, with body parts and feces remaining for extended periods after extermination. Unfortunately, because many of the cockroaches die inside the walls and in other inaccessible locations, this cleanup may be difficult.

The next step involves measures to prevent the cockroaches from returning to your dwelling. Identify and eliminate their entry points. Repair cracks and holes in walls, floors, and window and door screens, and apply caulking around any pipes that might provide a portal of entry. And again, probably the most important step in blocking their reentry is to exterminate the cockroaches in adjoining dwellings. This obviously requires either an understanding landlord or cooperative neighbors. Community action groups, if available, can also be helpful in such efforts.

Next, it is important to try keep your home free of the food and water sources that attract cockroaches in the first place. Restrict meals and snacks to one or two areas in your home, clean the kitchen thoroughly after cooking, store all foods in sealed containers, and wash all dirty dishes and cooking utensils immediately after use. Clean cupboards and cabinets regularly, do not leave pet food out overnight, and keep all trash in a can with a tight lid, and empty it daily. It is important to repair leaky faucets because cockroaches are particularly attracted to moist areas. Similarly, be on the lookout for condensation on pipes and other damp areas. Finally, do not store grocery bags, cardboard boxes, newspapers, empty bottles, or buckets inside your home because these are favorite haunts of cockroaches.

Finally, the issue of air cleaners comes up once again. Preliminary information regarding the particle size of cockroach allergens indicates that they are carried predominantly on large particles, much like dust mite allergens. If that information is correct, it is unlikely that air cleaners will make a significant difference for people with cockroach allergy, and I would therefore not recommend their routine use at the present time for cockroach control.

As a last resort, people with extreme symptoms may find relief only by moving to a new dwelling. I have taken care of several patients with severe asthma and cockroach allergy for whom we could seem to make no difference with the steps listed above. They were in housing projects where it seemed impossible to clean up a single dwelling in spite of significant effort, probably because the surrounding units were so completely infested. After much struggle, these patients obtained new housing and had dramatic improvement. So although I would certainly consider this a last resort, it may be reasonable in occasional cases.

Hopefully, this information will help to reduce cockroach exposure significantly in most homes. Future research will undoubtedly provide the means to deal more effectively with this difficult problem. In the meantime, the strategy for cockroach control relies on aggressive extermination, meticulous cleaning, and careful attention to the things in our homes which permit cockroaches to enter and encourage them to prosper.

CHAPTER 12

Mold Allergens

Molds are found in both indoor and outdoor environments. They are capable of growing wherever there is sufficient moisture and warmth. Several common molds produce potent allergens capable of inducing both asthma and allergic rhinitis. We are extremely fortunate, however, that most of the common mold species do not seem to do so.

INDOOR MOLDS

I will discuss indoor and outdoor molds separately because their control requires very different approaches. Indoor molds can be present on a year-round basis, although in most areas, because of their reliance on warmth and humidity, they are most prominent during the summer and fall months. Some areas, such as the deserts of the Southwest, are too dry to support any significant mold growth, whereas others, such as much of the Southeastern United States, are so damp that they encourage lively growth all year. Homes in those areas will obviously require much more aggressive environmental control.

The most common indoor sites of mold growth are the basement walls and floors, window moldings, shower curtains, and bathroom walls, ceilings, and fixtures. Molds in these areas will often be fairly obvious with a visible surface growth of a black, brown, or reddish substance. Some molds have a fuzzy appearance, and others are flat and smooth. Most give off a characteristic musty odor if their numbers are sufficient. Less obvious, but nonetheless very significant, mold growth can also occur on basement floors and in carpets, carpet pads, food storage areas, garbage containers, decaying upholstery and foam rubber, leather goods, house plants, and virtually any other area with sufficient moisture. The humidifiers and vaporizers that I warned you about with regard to dust mites can also harbor molds, particularly if they are not cleaned regularly. Cases studies have reported huge doses of mold allergen being sprayed into patients' homes (and noses and lungs) by contaminated humidifiers. Finally, contaminated air conditioners or air conditioner drip pans can also disseminate molds through a home.

Environmental control of indoor molds requires several important steps. First, you must eliminate mold breeding grounds whenever possible. When that is not feasible, attempt to inhibit their growth by lowering the humidity, and eliminate them by using fungicides (cleaning products that kill molds on contact) wherever you suspect growth. I will stress throughout that you have to be a detective to identify the molds in your home. Although some sites of mold growth are obvious, you will locate others only with considerable vigilance. Always be on the lookout for damp or unclean areas.

Therefore the first step in mold control must include an effort to locate and remove any sites of mold growth in your home. The most likely removable items would be old carpets, mattresses, or furniture. The carpets most likely to be contaminated are those in the basement and bathroom, especially those that have suffered prior water damage. It can be extremely difficult to kill the molds in these carpets (and carpet pads) because it may not be possible to get them sufficiently dry. You will have to remove such carpets. As a general rule, you should get rid of all carpets in the basement and bathrooms as well as any other rug that has a musty smell or which has had water damage.

It has commonly been recommended that you remove house plants from your home if you have mold allergy. Although it is true that molds can grow in the soil of potted plants, it is doubtful that they release allergens in quantities sufficient to cause problems for most people. Further, it has even been shown that house plants may help to clean the air of many pollutants and may therefore be beneficial. However, in large numbers plants may significantly increase indoor humidity and thereby contribute to mold growth. As a compromise, it is probably a good idea to remove plants from the bedroom and keep them in only moderate numbers elsewhere. And if your symptoms persist, you might need to get rid of them altogether.

Next, clean thoroughly all areas where mold growth is visible or where there is even a suspicion of it. Again, bathrooms and basements are the most likely problem areas, but inspect your kitchen, laundry room, and even your bedrooms. You should be particularly suspicious of areas that seem damp or moist, especially where there has been a leaky roof or basement or other source of water damage.

To kill molds, you can purchase specific fungicides or use a dilute mix of water and chlorine bleach (one cup of bleach mixed with ten cups of water). Once they are completely clean, go over problem areas again weekly, even if no mold growth is visible. In addition to walls and ceilings, pay close attention to tile, grout, window moldings, bathroom fixtures, shower curtains, and the areas behind toilets and sinks which tend to accumulate moisture. You can clean most shower curtains, although some may be so moldy that you will have to replace them. An effective way to rid a shower curtain of mold growth is to run it through the washing machine on a hot cycle with a few old towels, detergent, and a cup of bleach—it really works!

As I mentioned above, humidifiers and vaporizers can be a problem if you do not maintain them adequately. Room units are most problematic and, if you must use them, clean them thoroughly every day. Check central units, and clean them regularly. Similarly, air conditioners can become contaminated with molds, so you should clean their filters frequently and spray them with an aerosol mold killer if you detect any musty odor.

Overall, the single most important step for controlling indoor molds is to keep the humidity at a reasonable level. You can generally accomplish this with dehumidifiers, air conditioners,

and exhaust fans, as well as any other available means of aug-
menting ventilation. Further, avoid extra moisture, such as that
which humidifiers or vaporizers provide. It can be very helpful to
purchase a gauge to keep tabs on the relative humidity in your
home. You should attempt to keep the level below 50 percent at
all times. A level of 35 or 40 percent would be even better, but
this may not be possible in some geographical regions.

If you have a problem with excessive moisture in your
home, you will be amazed at the difference a dehumidifier can
make. These machines can pull a tremendous amount of water
out of the environment, especially in a basement during the
summer months. They can also be surprisingly helpful even in
the absence of any obvious problem with excessive moisture. I
view them as one of the more useful purchases that you can
make for your home.

Please be aware, however, that if you have a wet or leaky
basement even a powerful dehumidifier may not be capable of
keeping your home adequately dry. You must repair leaks and
block other sources of excess indoor moisture. This includes gen-
erous caulking, using waterproof paints, and maintaining proper
drainage systems outside your home. If all of these measures fail,
install a sump pump to help remove any excess water that might
accumulate.

As with dust mites, indoor mold growth has probably also
increased in recent years because of tighter home construction.
Make every effort to assure adequate ventilation. Particularly
important are exhaust fans to remove excess humidity from the
kitchen and bathroom. In addition, be sure your clothes dryer is
vented to the outside.

Before moving on to outdoor molds, I would like to cover a
few miscellaneous points regarding mold growth inside our
homes. In the kitchen, clean the garbage containers frequently,
and inspect the refrigerator for any excess moisture, especially in
drip pans below self-defrosting units. In your bedroom, be wary of
old furniture and mattresses, and keep an eye on your closet for
any moldy items (especially old shoes). If you have any concern
about an old mattress, replace it or encase it in a plastic cover. Air
cleaners may also be useful if you do not think it is feasible to
control the humidity adequately and remove contaminated
items. Surprisingly, Christmas trees can even cause problems for

some people who are allergic to molds. Although this may not seem to make sense, it turns out that whereas few people are allergic to the trees themselves, mold spores that are stuck to the needles may escape in large numbers as the trees dry out, causing significant allergic reactions in some people with mold allergy.

Maybe more than any other allergy, I find that people who are allergic to molds are at special risk when going on certain types of vacations. The situations that seem to cause the most difficulty involve hotels or homes at the beach and cabins in the woods. These areas tend to be very damp, and the accommodations are often closed up for extended periods during the year. Please be careful with these activities. Short of scrubbing your room upon arrival and bringing your own mattress and pillow covers, the best thing to do is open the windows and have your medication handy.

OUTDOOR MOLDS

Outdoors, molds commonly grow in fallen leaves, soil, thatch, moist debris, and on moist surfaces. They may become airborne spontaneously or with activity; you find the highest mold spore counts with activities such as lawn mowing, farming, and raking, which may lead to dramatic symptoms in some patients. Airborne levels of some molds reach their peak on dry, windy days, whereas others are more prevalent on damp or rainy days. Outdoor molds are seasonal in temperate climates, peaking in the summer and fall and then tapering off after the first frosts of the late fall or early winter. Outdoor molds may thrive year round in tropical climates, and in arid climates there may be too little moisture to support significant mold growth at any time.

Environmental control for outdoor molds requires both eliminating the sites of excess mold growth and controlling excess moisture around the home. Proper drainage around your home is critical. Keep drains and gutters free of blockage, and direct down spouts away from your house. Remove leaves and other debris that may accumulate regularly, and keep compost a good distance away. Ideally, your lawn and the house should not be heavily shaded.

If you are allergic to molds you should avoid or limit activities that encourage mold dispersion, such as cutting the grass and raking leaves. If your children have mold allergies do not allow them to play in the leaves. Farmers need to be extremely careful while plowing their fields or turning over their crops, as those activities give rise to prodigious levels of mold spores. If you must perform any of these activities and you are an allergic individual, wear a high quality mask at all times.

As I will discuss in more detail in the next chapter on pollen allergy, outdoor allergens can enter the home through open doors and windows and cause significant symptoms in some patients. It is therefore helpful to keep doors and windows closed and to keep the air conditioner running when mold counts are high. The same is true when you are driving or riding in a car. You can usually find information on current outdoor mold counts in your local newspaper.

Back to the vacation issue: if you have mold allergies you need to be particularly careful while hiking and camping in the woods, where you will come into intimate contact with a variety of molds that may be found in soil, rotting wood, leaves, and other similar superb sites for their growth. A high quality ground cloth may be helpful, but you should also consider preventative medications if you undertake such activities.

Avoiding molds successfully will therefore require your careful attention to both indoor and outdoor environments. Your strategies to reduce mold exposure must include removing sites of mold growth whenever possible, using fungicides wherever you suspect mold growth, and making aggressive efforts to reduce humidity and moisture. These measures can lead to significant reductions in mold exposure with dramatic improvements in many patients with mold allergies.

CHAPTER 13

Pollens and Their Control

As a general rule, it is much more difficult to control exposure to outdoor allergens, like pollens and mold spores, than it is to control exposure to indoor allergens. Short of enclosing yourself in a bubble, some exposure will occur no matter what you do. Still, various strategies are available which can help to reduce exposure to these outdoor allergens. Most of them are based on common sense rather than on science or research, so you will most likely have already employed many of them on your own.

As you will recall, pollens exist because they carry a plant's male genetic material; they act as fertilizing agents, which makes them essential to the survival of a plant species. Some pollens are carried from plant to plant by insects, and others rely on the wind for their distribution. Plants that rely on insects for fertilization tend to be brightly colored (to attract the insects) and to produce relatively few pollen grains. This means that pretty plants rarely produce enough pollen to cause problems with allergy. On the other hand, plants that rely on the wind for the dissemination of their pollen need to produce large numbers of buoyant pollen grains and hence are much more likely to induce allergic reactions.

I provided examples of a few common pollens and a review of the common pollen seasons in Chapters 5 and 6. The pollen of each plant has a characteristic appearance under the microscope which makes it possible both to identify pollens and to conduct pollen counts. With your naked eye, you may recognize pollens as the yellow dust that may accumulate on your car or other outside objects during certain seasons, especially during the spring.

As opposed to most of the indoor allergens, sensitivity to pollens tends to be quite obvious and easy to diagnose. Whereas someone with an allergy to dust mites usually experiences symptoms year round, the symptoms of people with pollen allergy follow a highly predictable seasonal pattern. These people may feel perfectly fine one week and absolutely miserable the next. The most common symptoms of pollen allergy are nasal congestion, runny nose, sneezing, and itching of the eyes and nose, particularly upon going outside. These are the classic symptoms of hay fever or what is more appropriately designated seasonal allergic rhinitis. Some highly allergic individuals will develop these symptoms within minutes of walking out the door in the morning. Others may experience asthma symptoms, and occasionally rashes will occur, particularly on the face as a result of direct contact with airborne pollen grains.

Environmental control for pollens is not an easy matter, particularly with regard to outdoor exposure. You should attempt source control, or the removal of the plants that produce the pollen, whenever possible. It might therefore be worthwhile to try to remove a stand of ragweed plants in a nearby field. Unfortunately, however, source control is rarely successful for two main reasons. First, most of us like to have trees and grasses—the main causes of springtime allergies—around us, and we in fact often do everything in our power to encourage their growth. It is ironic that many people move to places like Arizona to escape their allergies, only to begin irrigating their yard soon after their arrival in an effort to grow nice green (pollen-producing) grass.

The second reason that source control usually fails is that many pollens are capable of traveling great distances after they have been released. For example, even if you removed all of the oak trees from your property, there would usually still be enough oak pollen blowing in from surrounding areas to negate any benefit from the changes that you made in your yard. Even if you removed all of the trees from your neighborhood and confined yourself to that area, the effects would probably still be negligible because of the distances that pollens can travel. In fact, it is even possible to measure pollens on ships many miles away from land, which clearly demonstrates the enormous difficulty in trying to escape from pollen allergies.

A more effective step in environmental control for pollens, as I noted for outdoor mold spores, involves measures to keep them out of your home. These measures are practical and important because even if life is miserable outdoors, you should be able to establish a reasonably safe haven indoors. This is indeed a very real issue as one study showed that there can be high levels of grass pollen inside homes during the pollen season if these precautions are not taken.

First, be sure to keep your windows and doors closed at all times. To get an idea of how much outside air enters your home through an open door or window, think how cold your house gets when a door or a window is left open for even a few minutes during the winter. The same holds true during warmer weather except that the air is laden with pollen and mold spores instead of cold. One patient recently told me that sleeping with her window closed helped her allergies a great deal at night but that she was still very congested when she was inside during the day. When I questioned her further, I found that she would leave the door open most of the day to "air out the house." Unfortunately, while the house was getting aired out the pollen was getting aired in! She felt much better once she kept the door closed.

In place of open doors and windows, air conditioners not only cool your home but also help to filter outside air. They can provide great relief for anyone with significant pollen (or mold) allergy. These same rules apply to your automobile. You should keep your car windows closed and use an air conditioner if possible. Intense pollen exposure can occur while you are driving with an open window—I have seen many patients arrive at the office with their eyes nearly swollen shut after a ride in the car on a nice spring day.

For some people with severe pollen allergy, it may be necessary to wear a mask during certain activities in order to get relief. No one, especially children, is thrilled with this option, but it can help a great deal to reduce pollen exposure and allergy symptoms. So if medication does not control your symptoms adequately, particularly during activities like lawn mowing, a mask may be the answer. In addition, if you experience significant eye symptoms, wearing eyeglasses, sunglasses, or goggles will help.

Finally, some people may have to avoid certain activities altogether during the peak of the pollen season, especially on particularly bad days. In general, pollen levels will be highest on dry, windy days. In addition, pollen counts vary to some degree over the course of a given day. Research has shown that ragweed pollen counts peak during the late morning and grass pollen in the early to midafternoon. Particularly sensitive people may therefore be wise to avoid outdoor activities at these times.

In short, although your ability to control pollen exposure is limited, a variety of simple strategies may help to reduce your symptoms and medication requirements.

CHAPTER 14

Allergens in the School and the Workplace

It is not uncommon for patients to complain of problems with their allergies while they are at school or work. A number of common allergens might be encountered in schools, and an almost unlimited number can potentially be present in the workplace, depending on an individual's occupation. In this chapter I will review some of the more common problems that you might encounter.

ALLERGENS IN THE SCHOOL

Although most schools are relatively free of allergens, some may have high levels of various indoor allergens. A school's chance of having such a problem will depend on its age and geographical location as well as the presence of such things as carpets, furred animals, excessive dampness, and even swimming pools.

97

Schools with carpeting are much more likely to have a problem with dust mite contamination than are schools without carpeting. This is particularly the case in humid climates or if there is excessive moisture in the school. It is therefore very important to find out about the presence of carpets in the school if your child has significant mite sensitivity. I recently saw a young child who was having terrible problems with asthma while she was at school. I learned that not only was her classroom carpeted, but that she was having her greatest difficulty while taking her daily nap lying on the floor! If you think that your child might be having a similar problem, you should discuss your concerns with both the school officials and your doctor. If the problem is significant, your child might need to be shifted to an uncarpeted classroom, or it may even be necessary to investigate alternative school settings.

The presence of furred animals in schools can also cause major problems. Recently, a mother called to say that her daughter was having severe allergy problems because of dogs that were present at the elementary school! I was very surprised to hear that dogs were being allowed in a school, but I have since been told that this is not that uncommon. The mother had actually been fighting a losing battle with the school for some time in spite of the obvious nature of the problem. After I made several phone calls, wrote two letters, and visited the school, the school authorities finally agreed to keep the dogs away, although at least one teacher still refused to admit that the dogs could be causing a problem.

A more common source of animal exposure in schools is classroom pets like hamsters, gerbils, rabbits, and guinea pigs, which are actually quite common in preschool and elementary classrooms. Although they may be fun and educational, these animals are highly allergenic and can cause significant symptoms in some children. For children with only mild allergies, it may be enough simply to restrict direct contact with the animals and take precautions while cleaning their cages. Remember that cage cleaning poses the highest risk of exposure because the major allergens from most rodents are excreted in the urine. For those children with more severe allergies, the only option may be to remove the animals from the classroom altogether.

Another issue regarding animal exposure has to do with animal allergens that may be carried into the classroom by children who have pets at home. We have long been aware that cat allergen can be carried on clothing and other objects after contact with cats and that this allergen may then be deposited in other locations. A study from Sweden showed that rather high levels of cat allergen can be detected in schools where cats have never been present. Although no one has demonstrated yet that such secondhand exposure is capable of causing allergic symptoms, the researchers in Sweden did believe that the levels they detected could be high enough to cause symptoms in some highly allergic children.

Occasionally, schools have been found to have problems with excessive mold growth. This is particularly the case in schools with very damp basements or other moist areas and in schools with swimming pools. Just as in the home, you may need to do some detective work to find the sites of mold growth in a school. These sources should be eliminated if possible, and fungicides should be employed to further control mold growth. Again, the school authorities may need a great deal of encouragement before any action is taken.

Unfortunately, it has also been shown that many schools in this country are badly infested with cockroaches. Although the true extent of this problem is not presently known, it is certainly an issue in many urban areas around the country, as well as in some non-urban schools in the South where cockroaches are more prevalent overall. I have become increasingly convinced that this is a major clinical problem and that cockroaches may well be the most important of the allergic exposures that occur in schools. Since I have come to ask about this problem routinely, most children going to school in the city of Baltimore tell me that they see cockroaches in their schools on a regular basis. As in homes, aggressive extermination and cleanup will be necessary. It might even be necessary to consider sending highly allergic children to a different school, provided that you can locate a school without cockroaches.

Finally, a word about exposure to outdoor allergens in school: in addition to the obvious exposures that may come with gym class and other outdoor activities, the issue of open windows is as important here as it is in homes. Although it is not even possible to open the windows in many newer schools, the windows in older schools are often opened to let in fresh air during the spring and fall seasons—just the time when pollens may be at their peak. In the seventh or eighth grade I can remember sitting next to a boy who had terrible hay fever symptoms every time the windows were open. It seems that someone was invariably cutting the grass, and this poor kid would really suffer. No one ever thought to close the windows, which, in any event would have been difficult on some days because, like most older schools, there was no air conditioning.

So when a child seems to be experiencing allergy symptoms at school, many explanations are possible. You should pursue them by investigating the school environment carefully and then discussing your findings with your doctor. If you find a cause, try to get the school authorities to remove the allergen from the classroom or, if necessary, to place the child in an alternative school setting.

ALLERGENS IN THE WORKPLACE

Allergens are a significant occupational hazard for many allergic adults. Some of the allergens are obvious, whereas others may go unrecognized for long periods of time. In addition, as I will describe in subsequent chapters, there are many irritants and other non-allergic triggers in the workplace which may produce symptoms much like those of allergy. Although there are myriad possible allergic exposures in the workplace, I will deal here only with some of the more common and problematic.

To begin, it is important to note that all of the allergens commonly found in homes and schools can be present in the workplace. Furthermore, the same factors that influence the presence of those allergens in homes and schools are relevant to offices and other work environments. For example, carpeted offices are much more likely to have problems with dust mites, and older urban buildings are more likely to be infested with cockroaches.

In many newer office buildings problems with indoor allergens may be intensified by deficiencies in the building's heating and ventilation systems. These buildings are typically constructed very tightly to conserve energy, and most rely solely on artificial ventilation, which, if inadequate, may lead to excessive levels of indoor allergens and pollutants. In addition, molds can contaminate heating or air conditioning systems, with dissemination through entire buildings. I will discuss the full scope of this problem in Chapter 17, which deals with the sick building syndrome.

In addition to the common indoor allergens that may contaminate an office building or other workplace, many occupations involve exposure to high levels of specific, and sometimes very unusual, allergens. For example, veterinarians and animal care workers are exposed to extraordinary concentrations of animal allergens on a regular basis. In addition to the common animal allergens such as those of cats and dogs, laboratory workers commonly develop significant allergies to experimental animals like rats and mice. Even occupational exposure to cockroaches has been reported in researchers working in insect laboratories. Sensitivity to these animal allergens can make it difficult or even impossible for some people to carry on their careers, and, unfortunately, in some instances environmental controls cannot overcome the intense exposure that the work requires. At the very least, laboratory facilities should be well ventilated, and allergic workers should wear high quality masks whenever possible. In animal care facilities, special cage units have been designed which filter allergens more effectively from the air to protect the workers. In addition, in instances where a simple mask is not adequate, elaborate hood systems can provide much more effective air filtration. Unfortunately, these more sophisticated devices are cumbersome and too expensive for many schools and businesses.

Many different factory and manufacturing jobs have been shown to involve exposure to a variety of potent allergens. Some of these cause true allergic diseases, whereas others induce different types of immunologic reactions which can also produce debilitating symptoms, including asthma, rhinitis, skin disease, and recurrent pneumonia. Examples of such substances include various wood dusts, industrial chemicals, metals like nickel and platinum, and even some of the drugs that are manufactured in pharmaceutical plants. Food workers are at risk of developing sensitivity to substances as varied as flour, coffee beans, soybeans, and the molds that may be present in cheese, mushrooms, and malt. These reactions may be so severe that a worker may have to change occupations, and even then the symptoms may persist even after the exposure has ceased.

Farmers can be at risk for reactions to several allergens to which they are particularly exposed. Some of these are common allergens, such as the usual outdoor pollens and molds, which would be encountered by anyone performing outdoor work. Others, however, are unique to certain farm occupations. Allergic reactions to horses, cows, and other farm animals are quite common. Farmers are also at special risk for a condition called farmer's lung, which is caused by exposure to moldy hay. This condition is characterized by recurrent episodes of pneumonia, which can be extremely debilitating. Farmers exposed to moldy hay should therefore wear high quality masks to reduce their chances of developing this condition.

A final occupational hazard that may be of interest is called pigeon (or bird) breeder's lung. This is a chronic lung condition induced by exposure to high levels of bird droppings. Although I told you earlier that the feathers used in pillows and quilts do not pose a significant risk for allergy, these bird droppings can be very dangerous when they are present in high concentrations. This is rarely a concern for the usual bird owner, but it is a definite risk for anyone who cares for a large number of them. Preventative measures should include well ventilated living quarters for the birds and the use of masks by caretakers, particularly during cleaning activities.

Some occupations may therefore involve exposure to an array of potent allergens. If you suspect that you may be allergic to something in your work environment, you should discuss your concerns with your doctor. Just as important, if you or someone you know is involved in an occupation that is known to cause problems with allergy, address these concerns early on so that preventative measures can be taken.

PART 4

Indoor Air Pollution and Non-allergic Triggers

CHAPTER 15

The Importance of Irritants

It is a simple fact of life today that we are surrounded by an enormous array of pollutants and other irritants in both our indoor and outdoor environments. Many of these agents are known to have adverse health effects, and many others, even though they may not yet be recognized, may also prove to be dangerous. In this chapter I will review briefly the impact that irritants and other non-specific triggers may have on people with allergies and other respiratory problems. Then in the next few chapters I will discuss in more detail the specifics of indoor air pollution.

I will use the term *irritants* here to describe any of the noxious substances that pollute our air, including cigarette smoke, cleaning products, automobile exhaust, industrial chemicals and pollutants, and many others. Some are obvious and easily recognized, usually because of their pungent odor, whereas others are far more subtle.

Although these irritants may bother everyone to some degree, people with allergies, asthma, and other respiratory problems are much more sensitive to their adverse effects than are people without respiratory problems. The mechanism that underlies this exaggerated sensitivity is probably similar to the process of *priming* which I described in Chapter 2. As you will recall, priming refers to a process by which a person becomes increasingly sensitive to an allergen with repeated exposures. For example, during a pollen season, your allergies may seem to become increasingly severe, such that lower and lower doses of allergen may produce symptoms. Priming probably occurs as a result of inflammation that develops in response to your initial allergen exposures. As the lining of your nose becomes more and more inflamed, it becomes easier and easier to induce symptoms. At the same time, this inflammation probably also makes your airways more sensitive to the irritants in your environment. When allergies are quiescent or are being treated effectively, you may be able to tolerate an irritant much more easily than when you are having problems with your allergies. We frequently hear this from patients and find that people with poorly controlled allergies may be altogether unable to tolerate irritants such as cigarette smoke.

The same process occurs in the lower airways in people with asthma, for whom non-specific irritants are a major trigger of asthma symptoms. The devastating effects of cigarette smoke on the asthmatic airway have been best documented. However, if you have asthma, you may also experience adverse effects from many other common irritants, such as paints, perfumes, cleaning products, and a wide variety of outdoor pollutants.

In addition to people with allergic rhinitis and asthma, there is another group of people with chronic nasal symptoms who are particularly sensitive to irritants. These people have a condition called *non-allergic rhinitis*, meaning that they have chronic rhinitis but no allergies. There are several possible causes of non-allergic rhinitis, ranging from tumors to hormonal problems to the abuse of decongestant nasal sprays. The most common cause, however, is a condition called *vasomotor rhinitis*.

Although poorly defined, vasomotor rhinitis is a relatively common condition in which patients have chronic nasal congestion and, usually, significant nasal discharge. Even though these patients may look and sound very much like someone with allergic rhinitis, they test negative to all forms of allergens. Upon more detailed questioning, it will often become apparent that their major triggers for symptoms are not allergens but rather non-specific irritants or even changes in the weather or the level of humidity. These patients will therefore not react upon exposure to allergens but rather to things like cigarette smoke, fumes, and damp weather. It is more difficult to treat these patients than those with typical allergic rhinitis, although some will get relief from allergy medications, especially nasal steroid preparations. This condition is also frequently complicated by recurrent sinus infections. Allergists frequently see both children and adults with this sort of problem, and because their symptoms tend to be so persistent and difficult to treat, they may even be more likely to consult an allergist than are those people with true allergic rhinitis.

Finally, I would like to say a word about the influence of the weather on patients with allergic rhinitis, non-allergic rhinitis, and asthma. It has long been recognized that weather changes can have a detrimental effect on people with each of these conditions. For people with allergies, this may of course relate to the direct effects of the weather on allergen levels, particularly pollens and molds. In addition to this factor, however, there is clearly a more direct effect of the weather on respiratory symptoms in patients with both allergic and non-allergic rhinitis, as well as asthma. The reasons for this phenomenon remain unclear, but the fact remains that many patients know when they hear the weather report what kind of day they are going to have. Cool and damp days are most notorious for their adverse effects, but any major weather change will affect some patients. So whether it be hot to cold, cold to hot, wet to dry, or dry to wet, many people will experience increased nasal or asthma problems.

With this background information on the general significance of irritants, I will proceed in the next chapter with a discussion of the irritants themselves and the strategies to control them.

CHAPTER 16

Indoor Air Pollution

Most of us are exposed to a frightening array of both indoor and outdoor pollutants on virtually a daily basis. Studies have documented that many of these agents produce serious adverse health effects, and many others are controversial because of their potential toxicity. Indoor air pollution has been an area of active research for the past twenty to thirty years, and it is interesting to note that much of the concern about it came after the introduction of the tight, energy-efficient housing, which I have mentioned repeatedly in relation to indoor allergen exposure. The bottom line is that the energy crisis of the early 1970s, which largely prompted the development of such housing, has had a major impact on the health of the entire Western world!

People with allergic diseases and other respiratory problems may be particularly sensitive to the effects of indoor air pollution. In this chapter, I will discuss the common sources of indoor air pollution and the strategies you might employ to reduce your exposure to them.

PASSIVE TOBACCO SMOKE

There is little doubt that the most important indoor air pollutant of all is passive cigarette smoke. Its effects on health can be devastating, particularly for children with asthma and other respiratory ailments. Passive exposure to cigarette smoke clearly ranks as one of the most important preventable health problems in the Western world. In fact, it probably ranks second only to cigarette smoking itself!

Dozens of studies on the health effects of environmental tobacco smoke exposure have reached similar conclusions. In addition to being a carcinogen (cause of cancer), tobacco smoke is a tremendously powerful respiratory irritant. The data are most striking in studies of children, in whom passive smoke exposure has been linked to increases in both the incidence and the severity of virtually all respiratory disorders. These include asthma, allergic rhinitis, bronchitis, pneumonia, and infections of the ear, upper respiratory tract, and sinuses. Studies also show that passive smoke exposure even impairs lung growth in children and suggest that some children would never have developed asthma had they not been exposed to cigarette smoke. All children with asthma or any of the other disorders listed above will have more severe problems if they are exposed to cigarette smoke. Although high exposure is most damaging, any contact can be harmful and should be avoided. Child abuse would not be an inappropriate description for such exposure, and in fact, the courts recently came to that conclusion in the case of a child with severe asthma and his smoking mother.

There is also overwhelming evidence that passive smoke exposure can have very detrimental effects on adults as well. This applies to exposure in homes and in the workplace. Most concerning is now a general agreement that such exposure may be a cause of lung cancer in some individuals. This risk appears to be highest for the spouses of smokers. Many studies have now also shown that passive smoke exposure is a cause of reduced lung function and respiratory symptoms in many adults, particularly among those with underlying respiratory problems. Thankfully, these risks have finally been recognized and become more widely accepted, such that the government and many businesses have recently taken steps to protect the health of non-smokers.

It is a shame that it has taken this long and there is still a long way to go, but we appear to be moving rapidly in the right direction.

NITROGEN DIOXIDE

Nitrogen dioxide is a gas that is released from gas ranges, pilot lights, and many kerosene and gas space heaters. Since about 50 percent of the homes in the United States have gas cooking appliances, exposure to this agent is quite common. Although the data are not entirely consistent, several studies suggest that exposure to high levels of nitrogen dioxide is associated with decreased lung function, increased respiratory infections, and a variety of respiratory symptoms, including nasal congestion, eye irritation, and cough. Again, children appear to be particularly susceptible to these effects. Please be aware, however, that the exposure that occurs with the normal use of these appliances probably does not pose any health hazard. The greatest risk for nitrogen dioxide exposure occurs in homes using kerosene or gas space heaters or, even worse, in homes that use a gas oven for heat. This dangerous practice is unfortunately not an uncommon occurrence in many inner city homes.

CARBON MONOXIDE

Carbon monoxide is an odorless, colorless gas that may be released from a variety of sources, including gas appliances, cigarette smoke, and motor vehicles. Significant exposure can occur in automobiles or even in homes if there is a faulty furnace or if cars are left running in an attached garage. Although the typical exposures that occur in most homes and offices pose little risk, exposure to high levels may cause headache and drowsiness, and more extreme exposure can even lead to coma and death.

WOODSMOKE

Burning wood in stoves and fireplaces releases a variety of pollutants into the air. These include particulate substances (ash and other debris) as well as carbon monoxide and several other chemical gases. However, the potential adverse effects of woodsmoke on health are as yet somewhat unclear and are the subject of ongoing study and controversy.

As with all potential pollutants, the first step is to determine what levels may be seen in a typical home. For wood-burning stoves and fireplaces, this depends on the efficiency of the unit, how well the unit is ventilated, and how well the house itself is ventilated. Some stoves and fireplaces burn efficiently and are extremely well ventilated, and consequently they release very little smoke into the home. Others, however, leak badly and may create significant problems. Problems with leakage are generally greatest when the fire is being started and when it is stoked and when the stove is reloaded. If such leakage is combined with a tight, poorly ventilated house, pollutant levels will rise further, and the adverse effects of such exposure compound.

The true health effects of exposure to woodsmoke are still a matter of controversy, however. In one study from Michigan, the use of wood-burning stoves was found to be highly associated with the presence of respiratory symptoms in exposed children. This study led many of us to recommend a complete ban on the use of wood-burning units in the homes of children who have asthma and other respiratory problems. Subsequent studies, however, have questioned the validity of that report, and I have since tempered my recommendations somewhat. I still believe that any child with significant asthma should not be exposed to any avoidable respiratory irritant, including woodsmoke. Further, for anyone who experiences respiratory symptoms of any kind when exposed to woodsmoke, every effort should be made to discontinue wood burning. However, for those with mild, well controlled asthma or allergic rhinitis, I do not necessarily object to the use of a well ventilated wood stove or fireplace.

There is one other issue that deserves note. A couple of years ago a family in Wisconsin developed arsenic poisoning. After extensive study investigators discovered that the arsenic exposure had come from the burning of arsenic-treated plywood in their wood stove. You therefore need to be at least a little cautious about what you choose to burn in your stove or fireplace should you decide to use one!

FORMALDEHYDE

Formaldehyde is another gas to which we are commonly exposed. High levels, such as those found in biology laboratories using formaldehyde as a preservative, can be a significant respiratory irritant. The importance of low levels, which are present to some degree in virtually all of our homes, is a matter of controversy. A variety of products—including foam insulation, carpet backing, paper products, tobacco smoke, permanent press clothing, and the glues and adhesive binders used to make fiberboard, particle board, and plywood—release formaldehyde. Formaldehyde was first recognized as a problem when people living in houses constructed with foam insulation, which is made from urea-formaldehyde, reported symptoms that were eventually attributed to formaldehyde exposure. Although that type of insulation is rarely used today, there are obviously still many formaldehyde sources in most homes. Some mobile homes, which are commonly constructed with large quantities of particle board, pose particular risks with regard to formaldehyde exposure.

In addition to home environments, there are high levels of formaldehyde in some workplaces as well. In office buildings common sources include insulation, furniture, carpets, and cigarette smoke. Such exposure may play some role in the development of the sick building syndrome, which I will discuss in detail in the next chapter.

The adverse health effects associated with high level formaldehyde exposure include headaches, fatigue, eye irritation, throat irritation, and asthma. In addition, exposure to extremely high levels can cause pneumonia and even death. However, the impact of formaldehyde at the low levels seen in most home and work environments is not at all clear. To complicate matters further, research suggests, but has not yet proven, that chronic formaldehyde exposure may contribute to the development of cancer.

This is obviously a difficult issue. Here we have a very common substance that may or may not cause a variety of vague symptoms and even cancer. Clearly we need to be cognizant of the potential adverse effects of formaldehyde exposure. We should consider it as a possible cause of chronic respiratory symptoms, asthma, and even headache and fatigue, especially if someone is living or working in an environment with potentially high levels, such as a mobile home or a laboratory. Hopefully, more definitive studies will help to clarify these issues in the near future.

RADON

Radon is another difficult and controversial topic. It is a colorless, odorless gas that is emitted from soil and, to a lesser extent, from ground water and certain building materials. Radon is actually a breakdown product of the radioactive element uranium, which is present in small amounts in most rocks and soils. Radon itself is therefore also radioactive, meaning that it emits low levels of radiation. We are all therefore exposed to some level of radiation on a daily basis. Although this is generally harmless, it is also well known that exposure to high levels of radiation is dangerous and that exposure to high levels of radon, as might occur in uranium miners, significantly increases the risk of lung cancer.

Over the past several years intense debate has raged regarding the potential hazards of low level radon exposure. Although a large scale survey of homes has not yet been undertaken, it is clear that most homes have detectable levels of radon and that some homes have extremely high levels. These high levels are most often seen in homes that have been constructed over granite that is rich in radium. The radon gas diffuses through the ground into basements and crawl spaces and then enters the rest of the house. It appears that certain geographical areas are particularly associated with high radon levels. One such region is called the Reading Prong, which is a geological formation in eastern Pennsylvania, New Jersey, and Maryland.

As stated, exposure to high radon levels among uranium miners has clearly been associated with an increased risk of developing lung cancer. The next logical question, regarding the risk of exposure to lower levels in homes, is as yet unanswered. There is some evidence, however, that such exposure may be associated with a slightly increased risk of lung cancer and that the combination of radon exposure and cigarette smoking may pose additive risks. Most experts therefore recommend that radon levels in homes be measured to assess the possible risk even though exact guidelines as to what levels should be considered safe or unsafe are as yet lacking. This situation is even more difficult, however, in that we are even more limited in our ability to control exposure to this ubiquitous agent. Read on for possible solutions.

CONTROLLING INDOOR AIR POLLUTION

As with the control of indoor allergens, there are two general strategies for the control of indoor air pollution: you can either remove the sources of the pollutants or attempt to remove the pollutants themselves. Here I would like to provide some examples of how you might employ these strategies in your home.

First and foremost, do not permit cigarette smoking anywhere in your home or office. Many people will limit smoking to one area or another in an effort to try to protect a family member with asthma or some other respiratory problem. Although this is better than nothing, it is an inadequate and unacceptable approach. Since cigarette smoke travels widely within a home, *any* smoking indoors poses a hazard to the entire family. By the same token, smoking in the car, even with an open window, is unacceptable. Finally, I would argue strongly for the complete elimination of smoking from all offices, schools, restaurants, and other public places. Recent advances in this direction are most encouraging.

Gas stoves are another possible source of indoor air pollution. It is important that they be adjusted to burn efficiently and that they be ventilated to the outside if possible. You should never use them for heating purposes. Similarly, you should vent gas and kerosene space heaters to the outside if you must use them. And on a related note—never leave your car idling in an attached garage.

To reduce exposure to formaldehyde, you may need to remove its sources or else seal them to prevent release. As for all pollutants, increased ventilation will be beneficial. You can open doors and windows and use exhaust fans when they are available. In addition, keeping your indoor humidity levels low will help to reduce the emission of formaldehyde from particle board (in addition to helping to reduce mite and mold growth!).

To limit your exposure to other fumes and irritants, it is important to carefully store and apply chemicals such as paints, varnishes, and pesticides. Use them only in well ventilated areas.

Finally, consider having your home tested for radon. Testing kits cost about twenty dollars. Be sure to choose one that has been approved by your state or by the EPA (Environmental Protection Agency). If you find that the radon level is unacceptably high, you can take several measures to help to reduce it. Seal cracks and other portals of entry, vent your sump pumps, replace building materials that may be high in radon, and maximize your home ventilation. In some situations you may need to use fans that blow the radon gas away from your home. Professional contractors specializing in radon control can install them.

For more information about radon and these environmental control measures, you can call your state environmental agency or the EPA at 1-800-SOS-RADON. For general information about indoor air pollution, you can call your local or state health department or the EPA at 1-800-835-6700.

SUMMARY

Indoor air pollution poses many serious health risks and, unfortunately, appears to be an ever increasing problem. On a more positive note, significant changes have recently been made to help reduce exposure to passive tobacco smoke. Further, researchers are actively trying to define these problems better and to devise solutions for their control. For now, we should all be aware of the potential risks, examine our homes carefully, and take measures to reduce exposure to those pollutants that are under our control.

CHAPTER 17

Sick Building Syndrome

Sick building syndrome is another very interesting and problematic topic that has received considerable attention in the past few years. Relatively little scientific information is available on this problem, however, and a great deal of controversy and confusion surrounds it. Sick building syndrome actually falls under a more general heading of building-related illnesses, which can be divided into two general categories. In a specific building-related illness, exposure to a specific, identifiable agent inside a building can be shown to cause a symptom or illness, whereas in sick building syndrome there may be a variety of symptoms, but it will generally not be possible to define one causative agent. In this section, I will provide several examples of specific building-related illnesses and then discuss the more general problem of sick buildings.

SPECIFIC BUILDING-RELATED ILLNESSES

Several specific building-related illnesses have been described. I mentioned a few of them in previous chapters on allergens in the workplace and indoor air pollution. For example, developing allergic symptoms or asthma upon exposure to a work environment with high dust mite levels would qualify as a building-related illness, as would symptoms of eye irritation or sore throat upon formaldehyde exposure in a biology laboratory. One large study found a specific cause for work-related symptoms in about 50 percent of cases.

Other specific building-related illnesses result from exposure to the chemicals used in copy machines and in carbonless copy paper and pollutants from outside sources, such as motor vehicle exhaust or dust from building construction. Biological (living or infectious) agents have also been implicated as causes of building-related illness. These include molds that can be disseminated from contaminated humidifiers or cooling systems and which can lead to allergic reactions or a serious lung condition called *hypersensitivity pneumonitis*. Certain bacteria may also cause building-related illnesses. The best example of such an illness is Legionnaires' disease, a bacterial infection that can cause severe, sometimes even fatal, pneumonia. Several large outbreaks of this disease, including the infamous one at the American Legion convention for which it is named, have been traced to air conditioning systems contaminated with these bacteria.

Another specific building-related problem of great concern is caused by exposure to asbestos, which is present in the insulation of many older buildings. Although this does not fit the criteria of producing defined work-related symptoms, asbestos is a dangerous substance known to cause lung damage and cancer with prolonged exposure. This risk is well documented in asbestos workers, but the full extent of the risk from less intense exposure is not as yet clear. Because of these concerns, there is now a major impetus to seal or cautiously remove the asbestos from buildings in which exposure may occur.

SICK BUILDING SYNDROME

Although definitions vary, we will use sick building syndrome as a general term for symptoms that appear in a reproducible fashion upon exposure to a specific indoor environment, but for which no specific causative agent can be identified. In the building-related illnesses mentioned above, about 50 percent of cases had no definable cause or appeared to be related only to faulty ventilation. Because of its frequent association with inadequate ventilation, the term *tight building syndrome* is also commonly used to describe this condition.

The true extent of this problem is not presently known because of a lack of large, well organized studies. However, a World Health Organization report suggested that 20 to 30 percent of office workers may experience some manifestations of sick building syndrome and that up to 30 percent of new and refurbished buildings may pose a risk for it. Although I would be hesitant to accept completely numbers as high as those until further studies are done, the problem clearly is a very common one.

Many diverse symptoms have been described in association with sick building syndrome. These include eye and throat irritation, nasal congestion, headache, fatigue, drowsiness, dizziness, poor attention span, burning chest, dry cough, and sometimes dry skin or a rash. These symptoms, which may occur alone or in combination, tend to intensify over the course of a work day and then remit away from the work environment. They are more common among women, and they tend to affect groups of co-workers. In addition, stress-related factors, such as a heavy work load or strained relationships with co-workers or supervisors, commonly exacerbate the symptoms. The diagnosis of sick building syndrome is based on the presence of these symptoms in the absence of any identifiable building-related illness or other specific diagnosis. The symptoms are generally not accompanied by any physical signs of illness, and no laboratory tests have been useful, aside from those used to rule out other conditions.

Several specific building characteristics have been associated with an increased risk for the development of sick building syndrome. Artificial ventilation appears to be the most significant. One British study evaluated many of the symptoms listed above in relation to the type of ventilation in the subjects' work environments. All of the symptoms were more common in people working in buildings with artificial ventilation as compared with people working in buildings with natural ventilation, suggesting that the combination of a tight, energy-efficient building and artificial ventilation may provide the greatest risk for developing this syndrome.

Other suggested factors include humidity (too low or too high), high temperature, and excessive exposure to artificial light. High noise levels may also contribute, particularly to symptoms such as headache and fatigue.

Detailed studies in many buildings in which outbreaks of this syndrome have occurred have tried to identify specific pollutants or chemical agents that might be playing a causative role. In some buildings, high levels of formaldehyde or other specific chemicals apppear to be the culprits, whereas in others the symptoms have been attributed to environmental tobacco smoke. In most cases, however, the studies have not been fruitful aside from demonstrating that the symptoms are commonly associated with tight buildings and inadequate ventilation. Thus, although it is certainly logical to assume that sick building syndrome results from exposure to specific substances that accumulate in these poorly ventilated buildings, we are currently unable to identify the causative agents in most cases.

A final issue relates to the possible role of psychological factors in some patients. It is clear that stress, psychiatric illness, or even a general dissatisfaction with work might lead to some of the same symptoms seen in sick building syndrome. This is particularly problematic since there are no specific diagnostic tests for the syndrome. The possible contribution of emotional or psychological factors must therefore always be considered in evaluating patients with work-related symptoms.

When the diagnosis of a specific building-related illness or sick building syndrome is suspected, particularly if there appears to be a cluster of cases, it is imperative that authorities make an effort to determine possible causes. Once they have ruled out obvious factors, they may require consultation with both medical experts and specialists in building design and ventilation. In addition to medical evaluations, they may need to use a process of building diagnostics, which typically includes measurements of both ventilation and specific indoor air pollutants. These building evaluations can be accomplished through either public (government) or private channels. With luck, a specific cause that can be remedied will be identified.

SUMMARY

Building-related illnesses are common and important. Some are classified as specific building-related illnesses because they have been shown to be caused by a defined etiologic agent, such as chemical gases, molds, or bacteria. Others are classified as sick building syndrome, in which there is usually no identifiable etiologic agent but often an association with tight, energy-efficient buildings with artificial ventilation. The whole idea of sick building syndrome is obviously a difficult one. It is clear that the condition is quite common and that when present, it may severely impair work performance and office productivity. When it is suspected, patients must be carefully evaluated and a process of building diagnostics initiated to seek possible etiologies.

CHAPTER 18

Environmental Illness and Multiple Chemical Sensitivity

The terms *environmental illness* and *multiple chemical sensitivity* refer to conditions in which patients are said to be sensitive to a wide variety of foods and chemicals in their diet and environment. These conditions have also been called *twentieth century disease* because affected patients are said to react to the wide array of chemicals that have entered our world in this century. As I will describe, the techniques that are commonly used to diagnose and treat these disorders differ widely from those of traditional allergy and have not been fully accepted by most specialists in allergy and immunology.

Patients with environmental illness are usually said to be sensitive to a multitude of substances. Some are typical allergens, such as foods and pollens, whereas others are chemicals such as food additives, water additives, perfumes, cleaning products, and formaldehyde. The major difference between environmental illness and more typical allergies lies in this sensitivity to common chemicals. Virtually every chemical substance known to man has been implicated in one case or another. Most patients with this diagnosis are said to be sensitive to a large number of substances and, because of the ubiquitous nature of these agents, their lives are often dominated by their efforts to avoid exposure to them.

The symptoms that have been ascribed to environmental illness are almost as varied as the substances that are said to cause it. In addition to respiratory symptoms like cough and congestion, manifestations include behavioral disorders, depression, chronic fatigue, learning disabilities, arthritis, urinary symptoms, and a variety of gastrointestinal complaints. Even schizophrenia has been called a symptom of environmental illness.

In addition to the complaints listed above, it has also been postulated recently that environmental illness may cause a malfunction of the immune system which has been termed *immune system dysregulation*. This condition is said to include multiple abnormalities of the immune system, primarily involving impaired antibody production by B cells. It is postulated to be the result of exposure to chemicals in the environment, often in combination with infection or stress. It is important to note, however, that the usual tests for abnormalities of the immune system typically give normal results in these patients.

The diagnosis of environmental illness is generally made on the basis of the patient's history and a combination of laboratory tests. Although these tests may include traditional allergy tests like skin tests or RASTs, the diagnosis often relies on a variety of less traditional tests, many of which have been deemed unproven or invalid by the American Academy of Allergy and Immunology. The most common of these are serial end point titration tests and subcutaneous and sublingual provocation and neutralization tests.

In the provocation and neutralization procedures, a test substance is introduced by injection, or in the form of sublingual (under the tongue) drops, and then any reaction that may have occurred is reversed by giving a second ("neutralizing") dose of the same substance. A positive test reaction might include symptoms such as headache, nasal congestion, nausea, fatigue, mood swings, and behavior changes, which are then said to be reversed by the second dose. It should be noted that these symptoms are highly subjective and can be difficult to interpret. For example, in the best study that has been published to date on this procedure (in *The New England Journal of Medicine*, August, 1990), it was reported that positive reactions occurred with equal frequency whether the test substance consisted of the active allergen or a placebo. Moreover, they reported that administration of a neutralizing dose of a placebo was just as likely to reverse the reaction as was giving the actual allergen. The authors of the report concluded that these tests rely not on science but rather on suggestion and chance and that their results should be interpreted with caution.

Both traditional and non-traditional tests of the immune system are also commonly used in diagnosing environmental illness. And in addition to these laboratory tests, special diets are often also utilized for diagnostic purposes. These diets typically begin with complete fasting except for special spring water, followed by the introduction of new foods in a specified sequence, during which the patient is observed for the occurrence of symptoms. Again, these reactions can be very difficult to interpret because of their subjective nature.

The treatment of environmental illness typically involves steps to avoid the offending allergens in both the physical environment and the diet, as well as the administration of allergens and other chemical substances by either injections or sublingual drops. Attempts are made to rid the home and the work environments of all exposure to chemicals. In the home, this often includes the construction of so-called "safe rooms," from which all synthetic materials are removed. These rooms are often also built with special air filtration systems to remove pollutants. In its most extreme form, some patients are even said to react to the chemicals that might be released from a telephone or a radio, so that even those common objects might need to be eliminated. Since most environments outside the home could also pose risks, the patient's activities can be severely restricted.

Dietary restrictions for these patients can also be quite extreme. Processed foods are generally eliminated, as are foods containing artificial coloring or flavoring agents. Only special spring water may be allowed, and at times total elimination diets except for spring water may be prescribed. Another common practice is to rotate foods in a cyclic manner such that specific foods are ingested for three- or four-day periods in a regular rotation.

The use of allergy shots and sublingual drops to treat these conditions also differs markedly from traditional practices in treating allergies. Even when standard allergens, as would be used in traditional allergy shots, are utilized, they are usually given in much smaller doses than those used by most specialists in allergy. The use of sublingual drops is also controversial, with little research available to support this practice. And in addition to the usual allergens, these patients are often treated with chemicals, including such things as formaldehyde.

To give you a better idea of just how debilitating this condition can be, I would like to describe a patient I saw a couple of years ago. He was a young adult who came for further evaluation of his condition, which had been diagnosed previously as multiple chemical sensitivity and chronic candidiasis (see below). His main symptoms were severe fatigue and depression, which had been present for several years. He had been treated with sublingual drops and medications for candidal (yeast) infection and had been advised to restrict his exposure to environmental and dietary chemicals. When his symptoms did not abate, he searched for additional ways to reduce his exposures. He ended up unable to work (on full disability) and spent most of his time isolated in a "safe room" with special air filters and with foil covering the walls to prevent chemicals from leaking into the room. His social contacts were very limited, aside from doctor's visits. When I went to examine him, he had to take cotton balls out of his ears, which he used as added protection from the environment. He refused, however, to take the cotton balls out of his nose when I admitted to him that I was wearing deodorant! Although he came with an enormous medical file that was full of supposedly abnormal laboratory tests, I was unable to diagnose any allergies or other specific immunological problems.

When these patients are evaluated by physicians outside of this field, many of them are found to have a psychiatric disorder. One study found that 65 percent of patients with a diagnosis of environmental illness had a psychiatric disorder that accounted some or all of their symptoms. In fact, most of these patients have been told at some point that their symptoms were of a psychological etiology. The unfortunate result is that many patients are not receiving the therapy that they truly need and deserve because they have chosen to pursue this alternative avenue of treatment.

Before closing, I would like to mention briefly one other topic that commonly comes up in discussions of environmental illness—the candidiasis hypersensitivity syndrome (also called *chronic candidiasis* or the *yeast connection*). Proponents of this syndrome claim that there is an overgrowth of a common yeast, *Candida albicans*, inside the body, predominantly in the gastrointestinal tract. This overgrowth is said to cause a wide range of symptoms, including fatigue, depression, behavioral problems, headaches, rashes, abdominal pain, diarrhea, constipation, and congestion, among a host of others. Treatments include special diets and medications designed to kill the yeast inside the body. This syndrome has been popularized by a book called *The Yeast Connection*. In spite of its popularity, however, the limited studies that have been done on this syndrome and its treatment have been unconvincing. Further study is clearly needed.

As you can see, even though I am a great believer in the importance of the environment to our health and well being, I am skeptical about many of the theories and practices related to environmental illness. This is not to say that these practices have nothing to offer, but rather that so many of them have come into question that the whole field becomes suspect. If you are inclined to pursue these treatments, I would simply encourage that you get an opinion from a traditional, board-certified allergist as well.

PART 5

Product Reviews and Miscellaneous Topics

CHAPTER 19

Products Used in Environmental Control

In this section I would like to review some of the products that are currently being sold for allergen avoidance and environmental control. Most of them were mentioned in the preceding chapters, but I would like to take this opportunity to describe them in greater detail. This can be a very difficult area for the consumer because although many of these products are marketed quite aggressively, they are not always marketed with complete accuracy. In fact, in some cases advertising claims are completely without substance. My recommendations here are based on scientific data whenever possible. However, for some products scientific information is limited or entirely lacking, and for those my recommendations are based on personal opinion. Please do not take any of these recommendations as the final word on any specific issue.

MATTRESS COVERS

Impermeable plastic and vinyl covers for mattresses, pillows, and box springs are probably the most useful and cost-effective products available for environmental control. They are the single best means of reducing exposure to dust mites, which are typically present in their highest concentrations in mattresses and pillows. You should use the covers as your first line of defense for dust mite allergy. In addition to dust mites, mattresses and pillows may also serve as repositories for other important indoor allergens. Animal allergens, for example, accumulate in mattresses and may even remain there long after the pets are gone from the home. Attempts to reduce exposure to animal allergens in a bedroom, with or without removing the pet from your home, might therefore be doomed to failure if you do not also use these covers. Further, both cockroach and mold allergens are found in high concentrations in mattresses and bedding.

High quality plastic covers significantly reduce exposure to the allergens contained within mattresses and pillows. This is critically important not just because these objects contain allergens, but also because they place the allergens in such close proximity to the respiratory tract. Even low levels of an allergen in a pillow or mattress would therefore be more likely to cause allergic symptoms because of the direct exposure that these objects provide. Every time you place your head down on a pillow you may be stirring up a small cloud of dust mite allergen (feces)! Although hypoallergenic pillows are of some benefit, particularly in comparison with feather pillows, all pillows need to be encased to reduce allergen exposure effectively.

Although comparison studies have not been done, it is likely that most of the covers on the market are reasonably effective as long as they have a layer of impermeable plastic or vinyl and a high quality zipper. The main differences among the various covers on the market relate to issues of durability and comfort. Some covers are thin and flimsy and will be more likely to wear out or tear. Others will last for years, and it is usually worth paying the extra money for the more durable product. Differences in comfort can be even more dramatic. Some covers are made of hard plastic or vinyl fabrics that crinkle, crackle, and make you perspire, whereas others are made of a softer plastic or a vinyl laminate inside a cloth or fabric shell. These are more expensive but are generally well worth their higher price, especially for pillow covers. For the box spring, the less expensive covers will generally be satisfactory.

These covers are available in many department stores and from the mail order companies listed at the end of this chapter. The mail order companies tend to offer high quality products that are competitively priced, so you will usually do well to look there as well as in your local stores. Some of the mail order houses will even send you samples of the different fabrics they use and will make custom sized covers if necessary.

VACUUM CLEANERS

This is a difficult and confusing topic for the allergist as well as the consumer, given the extravagant claims made by some vacuum manufacturers and their sales people. I will do my best to clarify the little that is truly known about the differences among vacuum cleaners and then provide some general recommendations. I would also highly recommend a review of vacuum cleaners which appeared in *Consumer Reports* (February 1993), in which allergen control is addressed specifically.

First, understand that no vacuum does a perfect job of pulling allergens out of a carpet. This is not to say that vacuuming is useless, but rather that the majority of the allergens are left behind after vacuuming with even the most expensive unit. In one study, the concentration of dust mite allergen was found to be the same before and after vacuuming a small area of carpet for an hour! This is somewhat misleading in that this does not mean that no allergen was removed from the carpet—all of the dust pulled from the carpet did contain allergen, and the total amount of allergen left in the carpet had to be reduced. However, the burden of allergen in the carpet was so large that the vacuums were not able to alter the concentration of the allergen, even after a full hour of vacuuming. There were no differences among the different vacuums that were tested in that study, but it would be logical to assume that a more powerful vacuum would be capable of removing more total dust, and hence more total allergen, than a less powerful unit. Whether this makes any real difference for the patient is not clear, however. It may be that the differences are negligible because of the tremendous amount of allergen present in many carpets.

The biggest difference that has been demonstrated among vacuum cleaners has to do more with what happens to the allergen once it has been pulled from the carpet. It turns out that most standard vacuums leak significantly, such that much of the dust and allergen pulled from the carpet is simply blown back into the air. Leakage may occur from the vacuum cleaner bag, the vacuum exhaust, or through poor connections between hosing and wands. Although most of the airborne particles that are released settle fairly quickly, the end result is still far from ideal—the person doing the vacuuming may be exposed to high levels of airborne allergen, and a fraction of some allergens will remain airborne and cause ongoing symptoms. And worst of all, much of the allergen that was pulled from the carpet ends up right back where it started.

There are several possible approaches to the leakage problem. First, if you are using a standard vacuum cleaner, make sure that the allergic persons are not present during and immediately after vacuuming. If that is not possible, have them wear a mask, and open a window to help air out the room. A more ideal solution, however, would be to prevent the allergen from leaking out of the vacuum system in the first place. If resources permit, you can do this most effectively by purchasing a vacuum cleaner that is equipped with a special filter. The most effective of these have a HEPA (High Efficiency Particle Arresting) filter, which effectively traps even most very small particles. These vacuums generally cost four hundred dollars or more. If that is not financially possible, an alternative is to purchase special vacuum cleaner bags and vacuum exhaust filters, which fit standard vacuum cleaners and help prevent allergens from leaking back into the air. You can buy these bags and filters in many stores and through some of the mail order suppliers that I will list later.

My usual recommendation regarding vacuum cleaners is to buy a reasonably powerful unit that will not cost a fortune and equip it with a special bag and an exhaust filter, especially if an allergic individual has to do the vacuuming. A vacuum with a HEPA filter is probably the safest system, and you should consider it if your resources permit. Please remember, though, that the best way to control allergens in carpets is to remove the carpets altogether! Although that may not seem to be an option now, you may find yourself spending just as much money on fancy vacuums and products to treat the carpet before all is said and done. I would certainly urge that you consider carpet removal, at least in selected rooms, before purchasing a five hundred to thousand dollar vacuum cleaner.

AIR CLEANERS AND FILTERS

This is another enormous industry that has been built on relatively little in the way of scientific information. The concept is so logical and appealing—"just use this filter or air cleaner to rid your home of allergens"—that these products have almost sold themselves. In fact, a large number of patients have purchased an air cleaner long before ever coming to consult an allergist. Unfortunately, although the cleaners will rarely do any harm to anything except your bank account, in many instances they probably do little or no good. In this section I will summarize the information that is available and explain why or why not these products may be worth owning. For more complete information and for specific product reviews, refer to two excellent articles in *Consumer Reports* (February 1989 and October 1992).

Air cleaners are available as either central units or room units. Central units are designed to fit into your central heating or air conditioning system. Some of the less expensive models (twenty to two hundred dollars) simply replace the existing filter in your system with a more efficient filter. Other types need to be installed within the system by a contractor and are considerably more expensive. Although both types help to filter allergens, the efficiency of different units has been shown to vary a great deal. Further, it is important to realize that only a tiny fraction of the allergens contained in a home circulate through the central heating system.

Room air cleaners are portable units that are designed to clean the air of an individual room or other small area. These products may cost anywhere from one hundred to more than five hundred dollars. They vary dramatically in their effectiveness, depending on the amount of air that they filter and the type of filter that they use. It is very important that you read the product information before buying an air cleaner to make sure that the filter's air flow will be sufficient for the size of room in which you will use it. It is best to find a unit that will be capable of exchanging (cleaning) the air in a room at least five or six times per hour.

A variety of filtration devices are utilized to trap airborne particles in these units. Some air cleaners employ HEPA filters. These are highly efficient filters that are capable of trapping even very small particles, and as such they are usually the most effective type of air cleaner. Their drawbacks are that they are generally more costly than other types of cleaners, and they require powerful fans which in turn lead to more noise and higher energy costs.

The next three types of filters all use electrical charges to trap particles. Electrostatic precipitators function by giving airborne particles an electrical charge, causing them to stick to an oppositely charged area inside the filter; "electret" filters use static electricity in the filtering apparatus to trap particles. Both of these are quite efficient, although their effectiveness drops considerably as they become dirty. They require less energy but may end up costing more because of the need to replace the filters frequently. Another type uses a device called an ionizer, which charges airborne particles so that they will stick to walls and other surfaces outside of the cleaner. They therefore do little to truly remove allergen from a room, and, while the other types of air cleaners do an excellent job of removing visible dust, ionizers may actually make a room look dirtier.

A final type of air cleaner uses a device to generate ozone gas in the air. Although high levels of ozone attack and destroy some gases and germs, these units have no effect on airborne particles or allergens. Moreover, because high levels of ozone are very irritating to the respiratory tract, some of these units can even cause a form of indoor air pollution.

The true effectiveness of these products for people with allergies is still not clear. A 1988 review by the American Academy of Allergy and Immunology indicated that no data are available to support their use and recommended that using them "in the absence of other forms of environmental control is not sensible." A more recent study found some reduction in symptoms in dust allergic patients using a HEPA filter, although the true impact of the filters was difficult to assess because allergen levels were not measured.

How should you use these products? First and foremost, you should only consider them after you have taken other steps to reduce allergen levels. These products are simply not effective enough to serve as a first line environmental control measure. Second, although they do help to remove cigarette smoke, you should never consider them as an alternative to sending the smoker outside. Finally, since they are likely to be effective in reducing the levels of some allergens much more than others, you should direct them toward certain specific situations, rather than using them in a generic fashion for all people with allergies.

For example, as I mentioned previously, dust mite allergen is carried on relatively large particles that settle rapidly after they are disturbed. Since an air cleaner can only act on the fraction of allergen which is airborne at any given time, even a very efficient unit would probably have little effect on mite exposure. The more relevant mite exposures occur while you are sleeping in contaminated bedding, sitting in an infested chair, or vacuuming. The mite-allergic patient will therefore get far greater relief from using mattress and pillow covers and eliminating carpets and upholstered furniture than from employing even an expensive air cleaner.

The situation might be quite different for animal allergens, however. At least for cats, we know that some of the allergen is carried on very small particles that may remain airborne for extended periods. This airborne allergen would be available for filtration, and an air cleaner might therefore make a difference. This is most likely to be true where allergen levels are not too high, as in a bedroom from which you have barred the cat. If allergen levels are too high, the air cleaner might not be efficient enough to reduce levels sufficiently. We currently do not know enough about the airborne characteristics of the other animal allergens or of other indoor allergens like molds to predict the effectiveness of air cleaners in reducing their levels.

One final thought before closing. If you are concerned about allergens that may have collected in the duct work of your heating or air conditioning system, you might consider buying special filters that can be fitted over the vents, especially in the bedroom of the allergic family member. Although we do not know how big a problem this is or how much these filters really help, they are fairly inexpensive and do seem logical. I am especially worried that animal allergens may contaminate duct work and hope that these filters might assist in efforts to reduce exposure to these allergens.

DEHUMIDIFIERS

Dehumidifiers can be valuable aids for people who are allergic to dust mites and molds. Although there is only limited information to support this opinion, there are extensive data to document the critical importance of moisture to the growth of these allergens. Therefore, anything you can do to reduce the moisture in your home has to be of benefit. In addition to using dehumidifiers, you should also include air conditioning, increasing ventilation, and discontinuing or severely restricting your use of humidifiers.

All dehumidifiers work based on the principle of condensation. A fan blows warm room air over a cooled metal coil, so that water contained in the air condenses on the coil. This water then drips into a reservoir or into tubing that runs directly into a sump pump or some other drainage system. Dehumidifiers differ in the power of their fans and in their water storage capacity. They are usually rated by the size of the area that they will dehumidify effectively. Most units can be set to run only when needed, and some even have built-in humidity gauges. Dehumidifiers are available in most department and appliance stores and cost from one hundred to five hundred dollars, depending on the size of the unit.

As I have mentioned, an ideal indoor relative humidity should be in the range of 35 to 40 percent. If you feel that your home is too dry, especially in the winter months, you might consider using a humidifier as long as you are very careful not to overdo it. This is particularly important if you are known to be allergic to dust mites or molds, in which case you should buy a humidity gauge to monitor the moisture level in your home.

PRODUCTS FOR CONTROLLING DUST MITES

At the time of this writing, two products on the market are designed to reduce dust mite allergen levels in your home. I qualify this because I expect that several new products will be introduced over the next few years.

The first of these products is a chemical called *tannic acid*. This product does not kill dust mites but instead works by breaking down (denaturing) the dust mite allergen. So the mites themselves live on, but the specific allergens that they produce are rendered inactive.

Although tannic acid has been available for several years, there is still relatively little scientific information regarding its effect on allergy symptoms. We do know that it reduces mite allergen levels and is safe to use. You should consider it in cases of proven mite allergy in which carpets cannot be removed, particularly in bedrooms. But you should use it only in conjunction with, and not in place of, the other mite control measures described. It costs about twenty-five dollars to treat five hundred square feet (two or three large rooms), and it needs to be reapplied every two to four months, depending on your local climate.

There are two other considerations for the use of this product. First, you can apply it to upholstered furniture as well as carpets. This potential use has undergone less study, but it nevertheless might be worthwhile. Second, tannic acid also breaks down cat allergen. Although it is ineffective if a cat is still present in the home, it might help to reduce allergen levels more rapidly after a cat has been removed. Its effects on dog or other animal allergens have not yet been studied.

The second product is a chemical called *benzyl benzoate*. This is the only true acaricide—a dust mite pesticide—currently on the market. It therefore differs from tannic acid in that it actually does kill mites. You apply it to your carpets as a moist powder, allow it to work for several hours, and then vacuum it up, presumably along with lots of dead mites and mite allergen. It costs about twenty-five dollars per room, and you need to apply it at least every six months, with some research suggesting that more frequent applications might be more effective. A foam version for furniture and bedding is available in Europe and may soon be approved for sale in the United States.

Although studies confirm that benzyl benzoate kills mites and reduces mite allergen levels, information regarding its effectiveness in relieving symptoms is also limited. A potential problem is that even though this product does kill mites quite effectively, it is still very difficult to remove the mite allergen from the carpet. My current recommendation for this product is much the same as for tannic acid: it is safe and will help to reduce mite allergen levels, but you should use it only after instituting other mite controls. And as always, first consider carpet removal before resorting to either of these products.

ANIMAL DESENSITIZERS

Commonly sold in pet stores and veterinary offices, these are products that are said to make cats and dogs non-allergenic. Some are lotions that are applied to the animal's coat, and others are shampoos to be used in bathing. At present there is no evidence that they are effective, and it is not even clear how they are supposed to work. I used to discourage their use entirely, but I have recently changed my opinion somewhat. Since it has been shown that washing cats may help to reduce the amount of allergen that they shed, it is entirely possible that these products work by the same principle, at least for cats. The question that now remains is whether or not they work any better than water. Personally, I will continue to recommend plain water until I am shown that these products have anything more to offer.

SUMMARY

In this chapter I have attempted to provide information about some of the products that are currently being sold for environmental control. Do not take my views as gospel. They should, however, help to guide you on a few important issues regarding both your allergies and your pocketbook.

Finally, I promised that I would provide the names and telephone numbers of several mail order companies that sell allergy products. Although most of the products I have recommended can be purchased elsewhere, these companies generally provide high quality products and are usually competitively priced. Their only drawback is that they persuasively market a large number of products, many of which you may not really need. Your doctor may have brochures from one or more companies, or they can be obtained by calling the number listed below (most have a toll-free number). I list them here in alphabetical order.

- AllerGuard
  1645 S.W. 41st Street
  Topeka, KA 66609
  1-913-267-9333

- Allergy Clean Environments
  241 East Clements Bridge Road
  Runnemede, NJ 08078
  1-800-882-4110
  Fax: 1-609-939-2442
  Email: prevent@allergyclean.com
  www.allergyclean.com

- Allergy Control Products
  96 Danbury Road
  Ridgefield, CT 06887
  1-800-422-3878

- Allergy Relief Products
  246-08 Jericho Turnpike
  Floral Park, NY 11001
  1-800-862-5155

- Allergy and Asthma Technologies
  P.O. Box 18398
  Chicago, IL 60618
  1-800-621-5545

- National Allergy Supply
  4400 Abbott's Bridge Road
  P.O. 1658
  Duluth, GA 30096
  1-800-522-1448
  www.natlallergy.com

CHAPTER 20

Strategies for the Prevention of Allergy

There has been a great deal of interest in recent years in designing strategies that might help to prevent the development of allergy, particularly in children. As I discussed in the second chapter of this book, the likelihood that a person will develop allergy depends on both genetic and environmental factors. Because the genetic factors are as yet out of our control, most work in this area has focused on the possible benefits of manipulating both the child's diet and physical environment.

Although the potential influence of infant feeding practices on the development of allergy has been a subject of debate for several decades, there is now considerable evidence that dietary manipulation in infancy can have a significant impact in this regard. For example, several studies have shown that breast feeding helps to reduce the odds of developing allergy when compared with feeding with standard milk or soy-based formulas. It has now also been shown that the advantages of breast feeding can be maximized if the mother avoids major food allergens, such as milk, eggs, peanuts, and fish, during the time of breast feeding. If breast feeding is not possible or if a supplement to breast milk is desired, there also appears to be a significant advantage to the use of hypoallergenic (low allergy) formulas. Although early studies suggested that soy formulas were hypoallergenic, we know now that this is not the case. Soy is actually highly allergenic, and the only formulas that are truly hypoallergenic are those in which the proteins have been broken down into small fragments by a process called *hydrolysis*. Examples of such formulas include Nutramigen, Alimentum, and Pregestimil.

The benefits of these practices have been clearly demonstrated in a number of studies. In one, a large group of infants with strong family histories of allergy were placed on one of five feeding regimens and followed through their first eighteen months of life. The best outcomes were seen in the children who were fed either breast milk when their mother was on a restricted diet or those who were fed a hypoallergenic formula. In those groups about 20 percent of the children developed signs of eczema during the study period. The next best outcome occurred in children who were fed breast milk from mothers without dietary restrictions, in whom about 40 percent developed eczema. The worst results were seen in children who were fed a milk-based or soy-based formula, among whom the incidence of eczema rose to nearly 70 percent.

In addition to these issues, there is also evidence to suggest that the early introduction of solid foods into an infant's diet may increase the risk of developing allergy. I would recommend that for the allergy-prone child, you withhold all solids for the first four to six months of life and withhold the major food allergens—milk, egg, soy, peanut, wheat, and fish—for the first twelve to twenty-four months. Although these recommendations may be difficult to accomplish, they can clearly make a difference, particularly with regard to the development of food allergy and eczema during the first few years of life. Unfortunately, however, these dietary restrictions have less effect on the development of respiratory allergy, and their impact on the development of all symptoms appears to decline after the first two to three years of life. Thus, it appears that for most symptoms dietary manipulations lead more to a delay in the onset of allergy than to true prevention.

More in keeping with the theme of this book, several lines of evidence suggest that avoiding inhalant allergens through environmental control can help to prevent the development of asthma and allergy. The first evidence in this regard came from studies suggesting that early exposure to certain pollens might lead to an increased risk of subsequently developing allergy to those pollens. These studies were performed by studying the relationship of specific pollen allergies to both the child's month of birth and the intensity of the pollen season during their year of birth. Although not all of these studies have been convincing, positive findings have been reported for birch pollen exposure in Scandinavia, grass pollen in the United Kingdom, and ragweed pollen in the United States. Although these data led to the important concept that early and intense allergen exposure might increase one's risk of subsequently developing allergy, their practical significance is more limited. For example, to make use of these studies, a couple would need to plan conception such that birth would occur in a non-pollen season. While such efforts would not be wrong, I do not believe that the evidence is strong enough to make this a major consideration in planning for the birth of a child.

The more important and practical information in this area relates to early exposure to indoor allergens and non-specific irritants. Extensive work on the effects of dust mite exposure in infancy has demonstrated that there is an increased risk of both mite allergy and asthma itself in children exposed to high levels of dust mite allergen as infants. In one long term study, mite levels were measured in the homes of a group of infants in England soon after birth. The children were then monitored until they reached the age of eleven. The investigators found that those children who had been exposed to high levels of mite allergen early in life not only had a higher incidence of mite allergy but also were more likely to have developed asthma. These studies suggest that some children would never have developed asthma had they not been exposed to high levels of mite allergen in infancy. Further, once a child has developed asthma, ongoing mite exposure is a risk factor for more severe disease and increased medication requirements.

Although most of these studies have focused on infants and children, there is also evidence that mite exposure later in life can lead to the development of asthma. This evidence comes from a series of fascinating reports from the island nation of Papua New Guinea. It was found that in one area of the island there had been a dramatic rise in the incidence of asthma over the preceding twenty years. Analysis of this phenomenon revealed that this increase almost certainly occurred as a direct result of increased exposure to mites, which in turn was thought to be the result of the introduction of wool blankets. This increase in asthma occurred in all age groups but was actually most dramatic among adult males, which points out an ongoing potential for the development of allergy and asthma given the right environmental conditions.

Preliminary studies have now also demonstrated similar risks for cat exposure in infancy, and it is likely that the same will also hold true for other indoor allergens. These findings have led us to recommend strongly the implementation of early avoidance measures for the major indoor allergens in children who are felt to be at high risk of developing allergy. It is difficult to know just how far to go, but at the very least parents should consider undertaking basic environmental control measures for dust mites, molds, and cockroach and should avoid having furred pets in their home. In my mind, avoiding inhalant allergens will turn out to be at least as important as dietary manipulation, as was evidenced anecdotally by the case of Joshua in the first chapter.

In addition to specific allergens, it has now also been well established that early exposure to cigarette smoke may substantially increase a child's risk of developing both allergies and asthma. Although it would be prudent to limit any child's exposure to tobacco smoke and other indoor and outdoor pollutants, this is particularly important for the child born to an allergic family. Once again, I cannot emphasize strongly enough the potential damage that can result from exposure to passive tobacco smoke.

In summary, you should consider both dietary and environmental precautions for any child with a strong family history of allergy. By reducing early exposure to major food and inhalant allergens, as well as to non-specific irritants, I believe that you can prevent allergy and asthma altogether in a few children and substantially reduce the severity of disease in many others. The implementation of such programs will require extensive public education and the involvement of health professionals at all levels. Several European countries are far ahead of us in this regard, and we would do well to follow their example here in the United States.

CHAPTER 21

A Look into the Future

Intense research is under way in all areas of allergy and immunology, and this will undoubtedly bring many benefits to the patients we treat. In addition, however, the future may also bring increased problems with air quality and a variety of other environmental factors with which we will need to contend.

Medications for the treatment of allergy and asthma have improved dramatically in recent years, and there is no doubt that this trend will continue. Many new drugs are being developed, including several that are designed to block specific components of the allergic response which have only recently been discovered. It has become increasingly clear that allergic reactions depend not just on the release of histamine, but also on a number of other steps involving a variety of other chemical mediators. It is therefore not surprising that just blocking the effects of histamine is not sufficient therapy for many patients. New medications designed to block specifically the effects of these other chemical mediators are being actively developed. We anticipate that some of these will provide added relief for many allergy and asthma patients.

Other new drugs that have recently been released or are in the process of development are versions of older medications which have been improved by making them either more effective or less toxic. For example, some of the newer antihistamines work much like the older ones, but they do so without causing drowsiness. Others block histamine more effectively or need to be taken much less frequently than the older antihistamines. Similarly, new steroid medications are available which are both more potent and less dangerous than the older ones. Research of this type will undoubtedly continue with the certain development of new and even better drugs.

Just how effective will these new medications be? Although they will surely enhance our ability to treat allergy and asthma, no cures or other magic bullets are in the offing, at least in the foreseeable future. It is interesting to note that it was once thought that antihistamines would put allergists out of business, or at least severely limit their need, but that was far from the case. The bottom line is that allergy and the allergic response are far too complicated to be solved with a single medication or even a group of medications. I therefore view the recent and forthcoming advances in drug therapy as significant but not overwhelming. Further, I am certain that these advances will not replace environmental control and allergen avoidance as the safest and most effective means of treating allergic disease.

Treatment with allergy shots has also improved significantly in recent years, and there is hope that even greater strides with this mode of therapy will be achieved in the near future. A great deal of research is currently being done to try to develop allergy shots that will be both safer and more effective. All traditional allergy shots are limited to a degree by a small but unavoidable risk of causing serious allergic reactions. The problem is that although shots will not be effective unless a sufficiently large dose of allergen is administered, allergic reactions will occur if too much is given. If successful, new research focusing on ways to administer more allergen with fewer side effects would therefore be highly advantageous. In the final analysis, however, I believe that these advances will be similar to those that we will see with new medications—that is, they will make treatment more effective but will neither put allergists out of business nor replace environmental control as the most logical first line of treatment.

With respect to allergens and the environment, I believe the future will bring both positive and negative changes. On the positive side, I am confident that we will continue to develop new and better environmental control procedures for all of the major indoor allergens. For dust mites, I expect that new and better acaricides will be developed. It is not unrealistic to think that someday these products could virtually eliminate dust mites from our homes. In the meantime, however, we must continue to strive to develop other techniques to help reduce mite levels. In an ideal world, this would include major changes in home construction, such that factors favoring mite growth could be reduced or eliminated.

I am also certain that new and improved environmental control procedures will be developed for other allergens, including animal danders, cockroaches, and molds. These may include better air cleaners, new pesticides for cockroaches, or even chemicals that will effectively degrade the allergens that cause your symptoms. Tannic acid is a step in that direction.

The ability to measure allergens in the environment has improved dramatically in recent years, and this field will also continue to advance. This will allow for a more accurate assessment of the allergens in our homes, such that more specific environmental controls can be implemented.

On the negative side, the changes in home and office construction which have added to our environmental woes over the past two decades will probably continue or even increase. This may lead to increased exposure to both indoor allergens and non-specific irritants. There is also no doubt that new chemicals will be introduced into the environment which will be toxic in one respect or another. Thousands of new chemicals are developed each year, and, although attempts are made to estimate their toxicity before their release, their true toxicity cannot be established until large numbers of people have been exposed to them. For example, although no one ever expected formaldehyde to have significant toxicity, many adverse effects became apparent after it was put to wide use.

With regard to allergens, any advances that we might accomplish in environmental control will also need to overcome the obstacles created by tight home and building construction. Further, our pet population continues to increase, and there is no reason to expect that this trend will change. I expect cats, which produce one of the most potent of all allergens, to become increasingly popular since they require little day-to-day care and therefore fit well with our busy lives. In addition, we will almost certainly discover new and different allergens in our environment. For example, although dust mites and cockroaches were certainly causing allergic problems for many, many years, they were not recognized as allergens until fairly recently. There are probably other common environmental agents that are also potent but as yet unrecognized allergens. Who knows what will come next—if we had been told fifty years ago that dust mites and cockroaches were major indoor allergens, most people would have laughed at such a ridiculous supposition.

On balance, I believe that although new medications and improvements in allergy shots will make the treatment of allergic patients easier, the challenges from the environment will continue to intensify. The optimal treatment of allergy will therefore continue to require close attention to the allergens in the environment and the implementation of avoidance procedures whenever possible. Even though advances in environmental control will certainly occur, it is likely that most of the basic material I presented in the preceding chapters will still be relevant for many years to come. Thus, I would encourage you to tackle these issues now because, even with the dramatic advances of modern medicine, no miracle cures are in sight.

CHAPTER 22

One Hundred Steps to Effective Environmental Control

This book has presented a variety of techniques that you can use to reduce exposure to the allergens and non-specific irritants in your environment. As a final reference, I would like to summarize them here as a master list of environmental control. All of the measures listed below appeared in detail in the text of the appropriate chapter, as did a stepwise approach to the control of each allergen.

DUST MITES

1. Encase your mattresses and box springs in plastic covers.
2. Encase your pillows in plastic covers.

3. Remove stuffed animals.
4. Remove unnecessary fabric items from your bedroom.
5. Remove upholstered furniture from your bedroom.
6. Remove carpeting, especially from your bedroom and basement.
7. Vacuum carpets regularly if they cannot be removed.
8. Use a vacuum with a filtered collection system.
9. Control dust aggressively.
10. Increase ventilation.
11. Eliminate humidifiers.
12. Dehumidify.
13. Place filters over your heating vents.
14. Use acaricides, especially on your bedroom carpets.
15. Use tannic acid, especially on your bedroom carpets.
16. Use an air cleaner.
17. Clean your heating ducts.

ANIMAL DANDERS

18. Find a new home for your pet.
If that is not possible:
19. Keep the pet outside if conditions permit.
20. Limit the pet's mobility in your home.
21. Remove carpets.
22. Remove upholstered furniture.
23. Keep your bedroom door closed.
24. Encase your mattresses and pillows in plastic covers.
25. Increase ventilation.
26. Use an air cleaner.
27. Wash the pet regularly.
28. Avoid certain activities (for example, cleaning and brushing).
29. Clean and vacuum frequently.

COCKROACHES

30. Exterminate aggressively.
31. Use roach traps and baits.

32. Clean up thoroughly after extermination.
33. Encourage your neighbors to exterminate.
34. Seal cracks and other entry points.
35. Remove water sources.
36. Clean your kitchen after cooking.
37. Store all foods in sealed containers (including pet foods).
38. Wash dirty dishes immediately.
39. Restrict meals and snacks to one or two areas in your home.
40. Keep your trash in a tightly covered can and remove it daily.
41. Get rid of old newspapers, grocery bags, boxes, and bottles.
42. Clean your cupboards and cabinets regularly.
43. Encase your mattresses and pillows in plastic covers.

MOLDS—INDOORS

44. Remove sites of mold growth.
45. Clean suspected sites of mold growth with a fungicide.
46. Remove carpets from your basement and bathroom.
47. Limit household plants.
48. Eliminate humidifiers whenever possible.
49. Clean remaining humidifiers daily.
50. Clean air conditioner filters and spray with an aerosol mold killer if musty.
51. Dehumidify.
52. Seal all cracks and leaks.
53. Buy a humidity gauge.
54. Increase ventilation.
55. Use exhaust fans in your kitchen and bathrooms.
56. Keep windows closed when outdoor mold counts are high.
57. Use an air cleaner.
58. Vent your clothes dryer to the outdoors.
59. Encase old mattresses and pillows in plastic covers.
60. Consider using an artificial Christmas tree.

MOLDS—OUTDOORS

61. Ensure proper drainage around your house.
62. Clean gutters and direct down spouts away from your house.

63. Remove leaves and other debris from around your house.
64. Avoid cutting the grass and raking leaves, or wear a mask while performing these activities.
65. Do not allow your children to play in leaves.

POLLENS

66. Remove sources if possible.
67. Keep your doors and windows closed.
68. Use air conditioners.
69. Keep your car windows closed.
70. Avoid certain activities (for example, cutting the grass).
71. Wear a mask if necessary.
72. Avoid going outside during the times of day when pollen counts are highest.

THE SCHOOL AND THE WORKPLACE

73. Try to find a classroom or office without carpeting.
74. Make sure that there are no animals in your child's classroom.
75. Beware of mold growth.
76. Exterminate for cockroaches.
77. Keep the windows closed.
Animals caretakers, laboratory workers, and veterinarians:
78. Maximize ventilation.
79. Wear a mask.
80. Use special cages.
81. Use air cleaners.
82. Farmers: wear masks, particularly around hay.
83. Bird breeders: wear masks, and maintain well ventilated quarters.

IRRITANTS AND INDOOR AIR POLLUTANTS

84. Ban cigarette smoking in your home, office, and automobile.
85. Make sure your gas cooking and heating appliances burn efficiently.

86. Ventilate your cooking appliances to the outside.
87. Do not use your stove or oven for heating purposes.
88. Avoid gas and kerosene space heaters.
89. Vent space heaters to the outside if you must use them.
90. Increase ventilation.
91. Reduce humidity.
92. Never idle your car in an attached garage.
93. Remove formaldehyde sources.
94. Seal formaldehyde sources.
95. Use and store all paints, varnishes, pesticides, and other chemicals carefully.
96. Test your home for radon.

If radon levels are high:

97. Seal cracks.
98. Vent sump pumps.
99. Remove building materials high in radon.
100. Install fans to direct radon away from your house.

Glossary
of Important Terms

Aeroallergen   An allergen that is carried by the air and which induces symptoms after it is inhaled into the nose or lungs.

Allergen   Any foreign substance that induces an allergic reaction, including pollens, animals, dust mites, foods, and drugs.

Allergic conjunctivitis   An allergic reaction involving the eyes, usually characterized by redness, tearing, itching, and swelling.

Allergic rhinitis   An allergic reaction involving the nose which can occur either year round or seasonally. When it occurs seasonally, it is commonly referred to as hay fever.

Allergy   An abnormal sensitivity to a substance that is normally tolerated without difficulty. The best synonym is *hypersensitivity*.

Allergy shot   An injection designed to increase one's resistance to an allergen by means of administering gradually increasing doses of the allergen over a period of time. Also called *immunotherapy* or *allergen injection therapy*.

Anaphylaxis   A severe form of allergic reaction which may include hives, swelling, difficulty in breathing, wheezing, and a fall in blood pressure. Anaphylaxis may be fatal.

Antibody   A chemical produced by the body to defend against a foreign substance.

Asthma   A condition that causes narrowing of the airways in the lung through muscle spasm, swelling, and mucus production. Allergies are a common trigger for asthma symptoms.

Building-related illness   A symptom or a disease that is caused by a specific allergen or other noxious substance found in a building.

Candidiasis hypersensitivity syndrome An illness in which symptoms are said to be due to an overgrowth of the common yeast, *Candida albicans.*

Dust mite A microscopic eight-legged bug related to ticks and spiders. It lives mainly in fabrics and is a source of the most important house dust allergens.

Environmental control A general term for any environmental manipulation designed to reduce exposure to an allergen or other irritating substance.

Eosinophil A type of white blood cell involved in allergic reactions.

Formaldehyde A chemical gas that is released from a variety of products, such as foam insulation and particle board.

Histamine A chemical that is released into the body by mast cells and basophils in an allergic reaction. It causes many of the common allergic symptoms, including runny nose, sneezing, and itching.

Immunoglobulin A general class of chemicals produced by the body in response to various outside stimuli. Antibodies are types of immunoglobulins.

Immunoglobulin E (IgE) Of the five main classes of immunoglobulin (IgA, IgD, IgE, IgG, and IgM), those of the IgE class are formed in response to allergens. Later, the interaction of allergen with these IgE antibodies causes allergic reactions to occur.

Immunotherapy See *Allergy shot.*

Irritant A noxious or annoying substance.

Late phase reactions A stage in the allergic reaction which occurs several hours after the initial exposure. The reaction is characterized by inflammation and swelling.

Mast cell A type of cell which produces histamine and other allergy mediators. IgE rests on the mast cell surface, and when allergen contacts the IgE, an allergic reaction is initiated.

Mast cells are located in the nose, lungs, skin, and gastrointestinal tract.

Mediator A group of chemical substances released in an allergic reaction to produce symptoms like congestion, sneezing, itching, cough, and wheezing. Histamine is the best known allergy mediator.

Multiple chemical sensitivity A condition in which patients are said to be allergic to a large number of common environmental chemicals and food additives.

Pollen A microscopic particle that carries a plant's male genetic material. Many pollens cause allergic reactions.

Radon A colorless, odorless gas released from soil and ground water.

RAST An acronym for radioallergosorbent test, a blood test that detects specific allergies by measuring the IgE level to specific allergens.

Sensitization The process by which a person becomes allergic.

Sick building syndrome A disorder in which a variety of symptoms are caused by noxious substances that accumulate in a building, usually an office building. A specific causative agent is not usually identifiable, but the syndrome is commonly associated with artificial ventilation.

Skin test A method used to diagnose specific allergies by introducing small amounts of allergen into the skin and measuring the local response.

Index

ORDER FORM

You should be able to buy *Taming Asthma and Allergy by Controlling Your Environment: A Guide for Patients* at any bookstore. If this is not possible, please use this form.

Taming Asthma and Allergy by Controlling Your Environment

A Guide for Patients

by

Robert A. Wood, M.D.

No cash or C.O.D.s please.
Make check or money order payable to:
Asthma & Allergy Foundation of America,
Maryland Chapter

Shipping & Handling*
$3 for 1st book
Add $.50 for each additional book
Priority mail add $1.00 to total

Quantity_____ @ $14.95 each

Total Book Price   _____
MD residents add
5% sales tax   _____
*Shipping &
    Handling   _____

TOTAL $_____

Name _____

Address _____

City _____ State_____ Zip _____

Telephone (____)_____

Mail order to:
Asthma & Allergy Foundation of America, Maryland Chapter
Chester Building, Suite 321
8600 LaSalle Road
Towson, Maryland 21286-2002
(410) 321-4710
E-mail: aafamd@bcpl.net
www.aafa-md.org